Citizenship Inclusion and Intellectual Disability

CW01431472

What happens when a group traditionally defined as lacking the necessary capacities of citizenship is targeted by government programs that have made 'citizenship inclusion' their main goal? Combining theoretical perspectives of political philosophy, social theory, and disability studies, this book untangles the current state of Western intellectual disability politics following the replacement of state institutionalisation by independent and supported living, individual rights, and self-determination.

Taking its cue from Foucault's conception of 'biopolitics', denoting the government of the individuals and the totality of the population, its overarching argument is that the ambiguous positioning of people with intellectual disabilities with respect to the ideals of citizenship results in a regime of government that simultaneously includes and excludes people of this group. On the one hand, its members are projected to become ideal-citizens via the cultivation of citizenship capacities. On the other, the right to live independently and by their own choices is curtailed as soon as they are seen as failing with respect to the ideals of reason and rationality. Therefore, coercion, restraints, and paternalism, which were all supposed to end with deinstitutionalisation, are still ingrained in services targeting the group.

In equal parts a theoretical work, advancing debates of critical disability theory, social theory, and post-structural philosophy, as well as an empirical engagement with the history of intellectual disability politics and the ways in which present day politics target the group, this book will be of interest to all students and scholars of disability studies, disability politics, and political theory.

Niklas Altermark is a researcher at the Department of Political Science at Lund University. His work focuses on ideas revolving around vulnerability, as a grounds for exclusion but also as a resource of critical theory, in order to understand the historical and present government of groups that are judged to be deviating. Altermark's articles have for example appeared in *Disability & Society, Pedagogy, Culture & Society, International Political Sociology*, and *Review of Disability Studies – An International Journal*. Lately, he has been engaged in the Swedish struggle against austerity measures striking down on people with disabilities, chronic illnesses, and mental health conditions.

Routledge Advances in Disability Studies

www.routledge.com/Routledge-Advances-in-Disability-Studies/book-series/
RADS

Disability, Avoidance and the Academy
Challenging Resistance
Edited by David Bolt and Claire Penketh

Autism in a De-centered World
Alice Wexler

Disabled Childhoods
Monitoring Differences and Emerging Identities
Janice McLaughlin, Edmund Coleman-Fountain and Emma Clavering

Intellectual Disability and Being Human
A Care Ethics Model
Chrissie Rogers

The Changing Disability Policy System
Active Citizenship and Disability in Europe Volume 1
*Edited by Rune Halvorsen, Bjørn Hvinden, Jerome Bickenbach,
Delia Ferri and Ana Marta Guillén Rodriguez*

Intellectual Disability and the Right to a Sexual Life
A Continuation of the Autonomy/Paternalism Debate
Simon Foley

Citizenship Inclusion and Intellectual Disability
Biopolitics *Post*-Institutionalisation
Niklas Altermark

Not yet published:

The Changing Disability Policy System
Active Citizenship and Disability in Europe Volume 2
*Edited by Rune Halvorsen, Bjørn Hvinden, Jerome Bickenbach,
Delia Ferri and Ana Marta Guillén Rodriguez*

Citizenship Inclusion and Intellectual Disability

Biopolitics *Post*-Institutionalisation

Niklas Altermark

Routledge
Taylor & Francis Group

LONDON AND NEW YORK

First published 2018 by Routledge

2 Park Square, Milton Park, Abingdon, Oxfordshire OX14 4RN
52 Vanderbilt Avenue, New York, NY 10017

Routledge is an imprint of the Taylor & Francis Group, an informa business

First issued in paperback 2019

British Library Cataloguing-in-Publication Data
A catalogue record for this book is available from the British Library

Library of Congress Cataloging-in-Publication Data
Names: Altermark, Niklas, author.
Title: Citizenship inclusion and intellectual disability : biopolitics post-
    institutionalisation / Niklas Altermark.
Description: Abingdon, Oxon ; New York, NY : Routledge, [2018] | Series:
    Routledge advances in disability studies | Includes bibliographical
    references and index.
Identifiers: LCCN 2017027239 | ISBN 9781138088313 (hardback) |
    ISBN 9781315109947 (ebook)
Subjects: LCSH: People with mental disabilities—Government policy. |
    People with mental disabilities—Civil rights. | Citizenship. | Social
    integration. | Biopolitics. | Sociology of disability—Political aspects.
Classification: LCC HV3004 .A55 2018 | DDC 323.6087/4—dc23
LC record available at https://lccn.loc.gov/2017027239

ISBN: 978-1-138-08831-3 (hbk)
ISBN: 978-0-367-43100-6 (pbk)

Typeset in Times New Roman
by Apex CoVantage, LLC

To Sofia

Contents

Acknowledgements

The process of writing this book has been less lonely than I figured beforehand. To a large extent, this is certainly so since it was written in a truly stimulating intellectual environment: the Department of Political Science at Lund University. Thanks to all of you!

I want to single out a handful of people that have been of special importance. First Ylva Stubbergaard and Anders Uhlin, who provided me with good advice and encouragement at crucial stages in the process of writing. My friend and intellectual partner in crime, Linda Nyberg: I am sincerely grateful to have someone like you in my life. I also got great comments and criticisms at various stages of the writing process; Jens Bartelson, Jens Rydström, Ted Svensson, Sara Kalm, Ivan Gusic, Mirjam Katzin, Rickard Andersson, Ulrika Waaranperä, Martin Ericsson, Catarina Kinnvall and Emil Edenborg, thank you!

Outside of Lund University, I have been stimulated and inspired by Susanne Berg, Caroline Hammar, Vilhelm Ekensteen, Cecilia Ekholm, Christine Bylund, Vanja K. Carlsson, Julia Bahner, and the activists of Grunden, among others. I also want to thank Dan Goodley for a stimulating conversation about the arguments presented in this book. The end product has most certainly benefitted hugely from that discussion! Petra Björne, although we may disagree about many of the arguments presented in the pages that follow, your combination of smartness and courage have taught me so much; thank you for challenging me.

I also want to thank the editorial team with the publishers of this book, in particular Claire Jarvis and Georgia Priestley, thank you for making this a very smooth and stimulating process.

Lastly, I want to hug my parents, who have always supported me, have a cold drink and long chat with my brother and sister, and sing a song together with my wonderful children, Edvin and Albin. My grandparents, Uno and Brita, your pride means the world to me. Mosse, I miss you. And, lastly, Sofia, this book is dedicated to you and only you know why.

Part I

Introduction

1   Post-institutional

In September 2010, the local paper *Sydsvenskan* (sydsvenskan.se, 10–09–01) revealed that a person diagnosed with intellectual disability getting support in a group home in Malmö, Sweden, had lived with his arms tied behind his back for the last 25 years, more than 15 years after the approval of legislation that granted him the same freedoms and rights of personal integrity as any 'normal' adult person. It had been almost 20 years since deinstitutionalisation had been completed and succeeded by integrated living and disability rights; he should have been a citizen. Still, a sock had been used to tie him up; it was a measure ordinated by several doctors in clear violation of the law. It was meant to protect him; it was said that he would hurt himself otherwise, although no one had seen him do so apart from occasionally scratching his ears. To facilitate the arrangement, he only wore long-sleeve T-shirts that could be strapped behind his back and tied together with the sock. There was a schedule for the procedure. If you are tied in this way for 25 years, your muscles wither, coercion inscribes itself upon the materiality of your being. The productiveness of power, in a very manifest sense, came to shape his body. (svt.se – 10–09–01; sverigesradio.se 10–09–02)

The most convenient response to this episode surely is to see it as an anomaly, the result of a very grave yet local implementation failure and as something that occurs despite the policy goals of inclusion, citizenship, and personal integrity. Sweden, after all, is commonly seen as a role model as regards progressive disability rights and services (see Race, 2007:23–5). Such sentiments also flavoured the responses of public officials. The manager claimed that she had no knowledge of the incident, and the responsible municipal politicians declared that the man had not suffered any harm by the procedure (sverigesradio.se – 10–09–02). Everyone insisted that this would not happen again and that similar practices were not occurring in other group homes; it was a rotten apple in an otherwise appealing fruit basket. To a certain extent, this way of understanding mistreatment recurs in the scholarly literature on intellectual disability politics, where standard responses to shortcomings may go along the lines of 'we have good policies but implementation lags behind' or 'if everybody just followed the policy template then none of these bad things would happen'. Such sentiments, however, cannot explain why the ideals of citizenship, self-determination, and independent living seem to fall short more or less everywhere they should be guiding disability politics (Mansell, 2010:11): they cannot explain the locked gates outside group homes which house people who have been granted freedom of movement, they cannot explain locked refrigerators owned by people granted the freedom to eat whatever they want, and they cannot explain the everyday practice of staffers deciding how many cups of coffee is appropriate to drink if you are diagnosed with intellectual disability. Indeed, they certainly cannot explain why it only took a month and a few days before a very similar case of a tied-up man diagnosed with intellectual disability was revealed in another part of Sweden (sydsvenskan.se – 10–10–06).

Rather than an anomaly, I argue that this example of decades-long perpetual violence is an expression of a certain mode of institutionalised politics which operates by producing included citizens whilst simultaneously upholding their exclusion: not anomalous, but symptomatic of how people with intellectual disabilities are today being governed. The coexistence of technologies which produce citizens and technologies that withhold their fundamental citizenship rights is a defining feature of the present management of the condition. The production of citizens shapes the individual to behave appropriately, to learn skills of citizenship that staff consider important, and to manage their own lives in accordance with ideals of how 'normal' people live. The undoing of citizenship consists of restricting individuals, by rules, coercion, and paternalism, because people of this group are simultaneously seen as deficient with respect to the capacities associated with citizenship. The rationalities of these two technologies of government are coexistent and recurring, in disability services and policy discourse, and their contours can be seen throughout the history of Western political philosophy. Although they do not make the headlines, the daily practices of deciding what disabled persons should eat, how they should spend their leisure time, whether they should be allowed to have sex, how many cups of coffee their stomachs can handle, and what specific blend of coercion, bribing, and threats should be put to work when they refuse to take their weekly shower, are, in essence, all expressions of the same mechanisms of concurrently doing and undoing inclusion and citizenship.

Thus, the problem that I set out to make sense of is what has happened *after* the introduction of citizenship politics for people with intellectual disabilities; what such politics is premised on, how the boundaries marking the sphere of inclusion are monitored and upheld, and how power is maintained and control exercised after inclusion. My response to this will consist of two related arguments that I will develop throughout the book.

First, as hinted at earlier, the new politics of participation, individual rights, and self-determination that emerged during the last decades of the 20th century did not mean that power was moved from public officials to persons with disabilities or that power somehow vanished to leave room for an unconstrained individual freely deciding how to live. Rather, the government of intellectual disability became something else: a way of governing that relies on both crafting citizens and continually monitoring and correcting their conduct, sometimes by brute force, in case an appropriate citizen fails to materialise.

Second, in order to resist this regime of government, we need to attend to intellectual disability, as well as the human condition more generally, as marked by precariousness; that is, we need to get rid of the idea that the defining characteristics of humanity are independence and autonomy fulfilled by capacities of reason and rationality. As will be clear throughout this book, the question of how intellectual disability is governed is interlinked with what we take intellectual disability to be. Against dominating medical and psychological understandings, I will argue that intellectual disability should be understood as an expression of human vulnerability, concerning how our bodies interact with the world and how these interactions are culturally and socially constituted to become knowledge, classification, and, thus, subjectivity. To attend to intellectual disability as an instance of vulnerability does not imply that this group is especially vulnerable but that we need to acknowledge how the persistent neglect of our shared vulnerabilities has been an underlying rationale in the constitution and government of this group. The last three chapters will mobilise this insight as a critical resource for rethinking disability, ethics, representation, and hence the division between 'able' and 'disabled' more generally.

Citizenship inclusion and post-institutionalisation

Now, I want to specify the research problem a little further and introduce some of my key concepts. In Europe and North America, the last three or four decades have witnessed fundamental changes to how people with intellectual disabilities are treated and targeted by social policy, changes that were very often tied to ambitions of deinstitutionalising disability care and that were dressed in the terminology of 'participation', 'independence', and 'self-determination' (see Bigby, 2005:118; Clement & Bigby, 2010:159). The overarching goal was to end 'exclusion', interpreted as the lack of integration, rights, and autonomy of people with this diagnosis. Central to this mode of politics is the concept of 'citizenship', which here denotes governmental efforts that seek to heighten the status of disenfranchised and stigmatised groups by granting them the equal rights and status as full members of political communities. Thus, 'citizenship' concerns what the demos of democracy is: who has rights worthy of protection and whose living conditions compose the intrinsic aims of governing; who is 'normal' enough, competent enough, and human enough, to be a citizen? Following from this, the re-conceptualisation of people with intellectual disabilities as worthy of social and political belonging will be called a politics of *citizenship inclusion*, the principle object of study of this book.

As I will discuss further throughout, the politics of citizenship inclusion is designed to protect the liberty of the individual against a state apparatus which has, throughout history, treated members of this group as lesser beings who are unable to make choices about their own lives. Although there are, of course, differences between national contexts in this respect (we shall return to the extent of these later in this chapter as well as in Chapters 5), the concurrent featuring of inclusion by means of citizenship and the construction of intellectual disability as a biologically anchored diagnosis of lacking intellectual capacities characterises present disability policies in liberal democracies. Hence, we see processes of deinstitutionalisation, socially integrated living arrangements, legal frameworks granting individual rights, and commitments to 'independent living' and 'self-determination', across national borders and in the work of influential international organisations such as the UN and the WHO. At the same time, the results are often considerably less rosy than the stated ambitions: people with intellectual disabilities are far from the self-determined citizens, participating and fully included, that the new policies postulate (see Bigby, 2005:117; Johnson & Traustadóttir, 2005:14; Tøssebro, 2005:197). First, in the sense that institutionalisation prevails in some places and that many countries fail to live by their own commitments to citizenship rights. But more importantly, I believe, in the sense that the new services and legislations of integration and citizenship continue to restrain people with this diagnosis. In this way, contemporary intellectual disability politics is both embedded in promises of liberation and disappointments of bleak outcomes. This is the predicament of the era that I will call *post-institutionalisation*, where oppression has supposedly given way to emancipation and freedom but where power still lingers and there is a widespread perception that emancipation has failed. The allusion to 'post-colonialism' is, of course, intentional: drawing on Spivak's (1995 in Kapoor, 2004:639) analysis of 'post-colonialism' as the failure of decolonisation, we may ask what the failure of deinstitutionalisation is; what kind of political situation are we facing and how can it be made sense of?

To answer this, I believe that it is absolutely necessary to reconsider two central issues concerning intellectual disability politics. The first one is what this condition is. As stated, the dominant understanding is that we are dealing with a biologically anchored diagnosis of deficient intelligence. On the contrary, and for reasons I will develop soon enough, I believe that post-institutional analysis requires that we see 'intellectual disability' as a social phenomenon, constituted by certain discourses and knowledge techniques and ultimately existing for government purposes. The second thing to reconsider is how we see the politics of citizenship inclusion as such. Policies stating 'inclusion' as their main ambition are often depicted in contrast to a history of oppression – of confinement, paternalism, and dehumanisation – where the new services and legislations are presented as a relief, emancipatory in nature, and as the outcome of the admirable political struggles of the disability movement. Yet underlying this picture is often a crude and problematic understanding of 'power' and 'citizenship' as determinate opposites; citizens have power over their own lives, and governments restrain citizenship in their exercise of power. In order to understand present intellectual disability politics, I contend that we instead need to understand 'citizenship inclusion' as a new way of governing that operates by constituting intellectually disabled *citizen-subjects* (Cruikshank, 1999). Citizenship inclusion did not replace state power but is an instance of it.

Reconsidering these two aspects – of what intellectual disability is and how the relationship between government and citizenship should be made sense of – represents a way of understanding how this particular segment of the population is ruled. This is what Michel Foucault (1990:part 5) called *biopolitics* – the central theoretical term that I will start my examination from. From this theoretical perspective, it is necessary to analyse the formation of intellectual disability and the politics targeting this group together. Hence, central to what will follow is a theoretical link: between how intellectual disability is constituted and how the governmental efforts targeting the condition are designed. Consider here Rose's (2006:133) argument that projects of citizenship during the past 200 years produced citizens who came to understand their status as full members of society in biological terms. As we understand the capacities necessary for citizenship to be linked to the materiality of the body – and in recent times to the grey and white matter inside our skulls – the inclusion of non-whites and females implied rethinking the biological basis of their cognition; citizenship status for these groups was premised on dislodging 'sex' and 'skin colour' from notions of cognitive capacities. The reason why the label of 'intellectual disability' cannot be dislodged from lacking capacities in similar ways is that the diagnosis is defined by 'deficient intelligence'. Indeed, as I will elaborate on in Chapter 2, the reason why the characteristic of 'deficient intelligence' was consolidated into a specific category and label was the need to segment individuals who were thought of as lacking the capacities necessary for citizenship. This way of constituting intellectual disability as a deficiency residing in the brains of diagnosed individuals, is – and has always been – an integral aspect of how members of the group are being governed.

In other words, the same notion of citizenship that provided the yardstick that classified inferior intelligence as a specific category of human beings is today figured as the vehicle of inclusion for this group. What intellectually disabled people share is the fact that their brains and capacities are perceived as different with respect to what is considered 'normal'. Simultaneously, the goal of inclusion is that they should be able to 'live as others', that is, as 'normal' people. Indeed, to be eligible for special services that should produce independence, one has to be considered as someone in need of help. As we shall see, post-institutionalisation is frequently haunted by such contradictions and conflicts between designations of otherness and dreams of inclusion. These emerge as the border between exclusion and inclusion is renegotiated, that is, when a group which has served as the outside mirror of humanist reason, autonomy, and independence is to be included by what seems to be precisely these ideals.

Ultimately, this reveals a link to how the defining characteristics of humanity are understood more generally. Capabilities such as 'reason', 'autonomy', and 'independence', are central to a conception of subjectivity that emerged with Enlightenment philosophy, a conception that has since dominated our thinking about what it means to be human. The classificatory category that we understand today as 'intellectual disability' consists in the failure to meet these ideals; intellectual disability is their 'otherness'. Thus, we may reformulate the overarching problem of this book in more theoretical terms: what happens *after* the Others of citizenship are to be embraced by the same ideals that produced their exclusion?

The need for post-institutional analysis

As is clear from the foregoing, this book largely engages with a theoretical problem, where my aim has been to contribute to discussions revolving around inclusion and exclusion, normalcy and deviancy, and citizenship and government, issues which are all located at the heart of recent debates in political theory. The fact that these are theoretical issues, however, does not mean that they will be removed from the actual lives of people with and without intellectual disability in my analysis. In this book, we shall for example encounter people who have been held back in their everyday lives in ways that would be deemed unacceptable had they belonged to any other group; we will meet support workers struggling to implement policy – each and every working day from 7.00 to 16.30 and from 12.00 to 21.00 (or from 21.00 to 07.00 if working the night shift) – and we will discuss in detail how present classificatory criteria are constructed and affects the lives of labelled individuals. Thus, although this is a work in the political theory of disability, the arguments are constantly putting theory into dialogue with the empirical matters of disability politics. 'Theory' here, is considered to be a tool used to reinterpret the world, to make us question our presumptions concerning how it functions, which, in turn, might pave the way for actually changing it.

Bearing this in mind, I want to add a few things about the contributions of this book. 'Intellectual disability' does not entail falling short of just any ideal but of the absolutely central ideal of humanity as characterised by reason and rationality. As I will elaborate on in the second and third chapters, our cognitive ability is often seen as a quintessential characteristic of humanity, fundamental to how human beings are differentiated from other living things and repeatedly stressed in Western philosophy as our defining characteristic. Paying attention to a group that is perceived as failing with respect to this ideal provides the opportunity to expose the limits of a politics that is fuelled by a will to include, inherent to modernity, humanism, and liberal democracy. As a contribution to social and political theory, thus, I argue that intellectual disability is a crucial case; the study of 'intellectual disability' provides a privileged position from which the inner workings of a model of emancipation founded on ideas of self-determination, self-sufficiency, and autonomy can be critically assessed (Clifford Simplican, 2015:3). A vital aspect of my analysis will be that intellectual disability contains the norm that it is separated from. Therefore, examining how we construct and govern 'deviancy' also entails that we analyse the unacknowledged norm of appropriate cognitive functioning that disabled people are compared to (see Goodley, 2014:26). This means that this is not a book about 'intellectual disability' but about the dividing line between 'normalcy' and 'deviancy' – a division in relation to which we are all situated. In this sense, the politics of intellectual disability is also 'the politics of all of us'.

As a contribution to disability studies, on the other hand, my analysis provides the first book-length examination of intellectual disability from the theoretical perspective of biopolitics. Carlson (2010:12) argues that attempts by critical disability scholars to destabilise notions of 'impairment' and 'disability' have tended to overlook cognitive impairments. In response to this, I would argue that 'intellectual disability' is pivotal to understanding the mechanisms of a disabling society, precisely because this particular condition is taken to be located at the heart of subjectivity: in the brain of the individual. 'Intellectual disability' is not just another category whose inclusion deserves recognition; it is, arguably, *the* group that exposes how the ideals of the humanist subject operate in politics that are geared to include (Erevelles, 2002:22); the group in which the governmental rationalities of citizenship are most clearly crystalized and in which the stigma directed against numerous others is implied (see Goodley, 2014:13).

Last, a cautious reminder. As is evident, this book entails a lot of critical discussions of notions such as 'citizenship', 'independence', and 'inclusion', that is, of concepts that were integral to the abandonment of institutionalisation. This certainly does not imply that I promote 'exclusion', 'dependence', 'paternalism', or any other remnant of institutional disability care (see Simons & Masschelein, 2005:209). I agree with almost everyone else writing on this topic that deinstitutionalisation and policies of inclusion were very much called for, and I fully accept that the services emerging after deinstitutionalisation have often meant better lives for people belonging to this group (see Bigby, 2005; Tøssebro, 2005; Clement & Bigby, 2010:25–27). Still, I do not infer from this that the present policies should be immune to criticism or that they, by merit of not being the harsh oppression of institutional confinement, are untouched by power. That deinstitutionalisation and citizenship politics were badly needed at that time does not mean that they marked the end of politics or the end of power or that they should imply the end of critique.

Structure of the book

To make sense of the politics of post-institutionalisation, I set out to tackle three distinct analytical tasks. *First*, starting from Foucault's conception of biopolitics, I will examine the fundamental linkage between intellectual disability as an object of knowledge and as a subject of management. This means making sense of how this condition emerged to make certain governmental responses possible and what this implies for how we should approach what intellectual disability is. *Second*, I will analyse the politics of citizenship inclusion, targeting people with intellectual disability. As I hinted at earlier, rather than starting from a certain conception of 'citizenship' or using it as a notion with a pre-established content, I believe that we must analyse how citizenship is made, or, more specifically, how citizens are made (see Cruikshank, 1999). *Third*, I will try to make sense of the possibilities of resistance against the present biopolitical regime and what this may reveal about the future of intellectual disability politics.

These analytical tasks provide the general structure of what follows. In the next chapter, I discuss 'intellectual disability' as a medico-historical phenomenon, where I argue that we need to understand this condition beyond an ontological separation between 'nature' and 'politics'. Thereafter follow the two main parts of the book – called 'Citizenship' and 'Resistance'. Part II is devoted to interpreting intellectual disability politics after inclusion, engaging with the history and present of intellectual disability in political theory (Chapter 3), how ideals of citizenship inclusion are discursively constructed by global and transnational organisations (Chapter 4), and how citizenship inclusion plays out in supported living services (Chapter 5). The three chapters of Part III aim to develop theoretical tools that can be used to rethink the politics of intellectual disability, engaging three separate instances of resistance and contestation. First, I will discuss how support workers resist ideals of citizenship (Chapter 6), then how activists with intellectual disability engage in a politics of representation (Chapter 7), and, last, how discourses surrounding prenatal diagnosis restrain and make possible different forms of contestation (Chapter 8). Thus, the second part of the book presents us with an interpretation of post-institutional politics, whilst the third part offers an analysis of how we can break free of its grip. Now, the rest of this chapter will present the theoretical starting points that shall guide this endeavour.

Theorising intellectual disability politics

The purpose of this and the sections that follow is twofold: first, I want to discuss some tendencies of intellectual disability research that my own approach is set up against and, second, I will present a number of theoretical concepts that will be central for my own investigation.

Consider again the central starting point stressed earlier: this is not a book about 'people with intellectual disabilities'. I do not believe that individuals labelled so have an essence, a set of common and knowable interests, or a unified voice that I shall make heard. I am interested in 'intellectual disability' as a biopolitical categorisation, and one of the purposes of my analysis is to denaturalise its existence by pointing out the political considerations that underpin it. This is akin to what Butler discusses as 'genealogical critique', in her case on the categories of gender. At the opening of *Gender Trouble* (1990:xxxi), she explains that

> a genealogical critique refuses to search for the origins of gender, the inner truth of female desire, a genuine or authentic sexual identity that repression has kept from view; rather genealogy investigates the political stakes in designating as an *origin* or *cause* those identity categories that are the *effects* of institutions, practices, discourses with multiple and diffuse points of origin.

Similarly, the focus of my analysis will be on how the condition of intellectual disability is constituted, that is, how it is *done*, and how people labelled with this diagnosis are being governed. This does not imply that I will seek to do away with 'intellectual disability' as such or that the differences that mark this group are, in fact, spurious or irrelevant. Rather, the project is to examine *how* 'intellectual disability' comes to matter by focusing on how the category functions and is targeted by politics of inclusion (see Butler, 1993:5–6).

In order to understand the need for this theoretical approach, it is necessary to first say something about how citizenship politics targeting this group is commonly perceived and how the history of the group is narrated – in social scientific research and more broadly. The problem of this book is set up against the background of a popular history of disability politics: the story of grim oppression which hard-fought victories transformed into citizenship and inclusion. We shall start by analysing this narrative before turning to discuss some theoretical tools that can help us break free of its grip.

Emancipation and disappointment

Intellectual disability emerged as a distinct category, in the form we know it today, at the end of the 19th century and was consolidated as a specific administrative category during the following decades. The opportunity to pinpoint people with 'mental deficits', provided by the invention of psychometric testing (discussed in detail in Chapter 2), formed the basis for the governmental regime that would dominate the 20th century. This regime entailed institutionalisation, eugenics, and an on-going search for the biological causes of lesser intelligence. Although the emerging welfare states came to develop along different trajectories, histories of institutionalisation and classification are surprisingly similar across national borders: institutional confinement developed, to varying degrees and in various forms, in most countries, founded on the dual logics of ameliorating disability and protecting society from the disabled (Walmsley, 2005:51; Carlson, 2010:42–3). It was in contrast to this world, the world of the institution, that intellectual disability policies would be reformed and take aim at citizenship.

The moment of inclusion did not occur overnight or precisely at the same time. Rather it consisted of a succession of changing policies, aiming to include the intellectually disabled in the citizenry in a number of Western countries and over a time span of at least 40 years. The process and ideas of deinstitutionalisation had arguably already begun in the 1960s, at least in the United States, the UK, and in Scandinavia (see Parmeter, 2004:9; Nehring & Betz, 2007:82). In successive steps, dormitories decreased in size and were finally replaced by group homes and other models of socially integrated living. At the same time, new policies made individual rights, participation, and an emphasis on self-determination and autonomy cornerstones of the citizenship status of people with disabilities. Different countries have their own milestones to narrate this story: the 1975 Education of the Handicapped Children Act and the 1990 Americans with Disabilities Act (ADA) in the US; the Swedish Omsorgslag of 1986 and the Law of Support and Service (LSS) of 1994; the 1995 Disability Discrimination Act and the *Valuing People* strategy of 2001 (Department of Health, 2001) in the UK, and so on. A number of cross-national efforts, such as the 1982 UN *World Programme of Action Concerning Disabled Persons* and the 2007 UN *Convention on the Rights of the Disabled* (CRPD) can also be seen as parts of this wave of efforts to include. These policies all seemed to cast themselves against a shadow of confinement, discrimination, and paternalism and instead promoted community living, integration, and independence (see Walmsley, 2005:52; Clifford Simplican, 2015:98). Although the process of deinstitutionalisation still is far from completed in many places, and that there are worrying signs of re-institutionalisation in some countries, the overarching idea of a movement, from confinement to social integration, is common in how policy developments are commonly interpreted.

The story of what has happened since is dual in nature. First, it should be noted that the politics of inclusion is understood as being a clear and important break with the past, often a source of pride which answers to the historical guilt of how people with intellectual disabilities have previously been treated. Simultaneously, as I have already mentioned, there has also been a lot of disappointment with regards to the outcomes. People with intellectual disabilities are still not equal and fully integrated citizens. On the contrary, members of this group lag behind in more or less every standard of living or socio-economic measurement scale there is (see Tøssebro, 2005; Clement & Bigby, 2010:160). Indeed, as Mansell (2010:11) notes, the recognition of a gap between ideals and outcomes of independent and community living has been prevalent more or less since 'citizenship inclusion' came to guide disability politics (see Cumella, 2008; Clement & Bigby, 2010).

This history of deinstitutionalisation, liberation, and disappointment is also ingrained in much of the social scientific research on intellectual disability. 'The lyricism of the cold monster' is what Foucault (2007:109) calls the tendency to start every discussion about power with the state, pictured as oppressive and reigning over and down on its people. A considerable degree of such lyricism is present in social scientific research about disability. Hence, the perceived enemy is the totalising institution that confines, forces, subjects, and constrains. Therefore the ambition – whether it be stated or implicit – of much disability research has become to guard the freedom of the individual against a vindictive state. In practice, this guarding often consists of measuring disability services against some pre-set standard used to localise failures (see Yates, 2005:75; Fyson & Fox, 2013). Often starting from a phase-based and instrumental view of policy processes (Hill & Hupe, 2009:5–8), a lot of research on intellectual disability takes the smooth following of regulations and rules as an unquestioned descriptive ideal (see Drake, 1999:25–9; Bigby, 2005). Indeed, social scientists and public commissioners regularly conclude that disability service personnel 'still' possess power and that people with disabilities are not 'yet' independent (Drake, 1999:90–1; Gustavsson, 2004:56; Larsson, 2008). From this perspective, any conceptual complications or discursive implications of these policies are effectively precluded. When it turns out that people with intellectual disabilities are not independent despite the stated ambitions of inclusive policies, it is interpreted as an indicator of disability services suffering from 'implementation failures', explained by the persistence of an institutionalisation mentality, lack of resources, or dysfunctional organisation of service provision (see Drake, 1999:91; Bigby, 2005:118–19; Clement & Bigby, 2010:32). According to this line of reasoning, if everything had only worked out as it was intended to, then public power would have been dismantled and citizenship granted for the targeted group.

Identifying paternalism and the neglect of legal rights has obvious merits. However, there are also notable perils, the main one being that there is a tendency to uncritically accept the present formulations of policy goals. An instrumental view on policy implementation that takes the link between emancipation and citizenship for granted can never detect if or how power is systematised within present disability services as something else than a residue of practices that our present policies have sworn themselves free from. Hence, there is a predisposition to answer questions formulated from the perspectives of administrators and politicians, where the focus is to facilitate organisational efficiency and goal compliance rather than to examine the wider implications of disability policies (see Mabbett, 2004:32). As a result, stories of the kind that I started this introduction with – of the tied-up man in Malmö, Sweden – are easily recognised as an exercise of power in violation of the law, an anomaly against a backdrop of good intentions. But this perspective will not help us see how this example is an expression of a systematised mode of government. Nor can it help us understand that government also may operate by actively shaping people to become citizens *in accordance* with the ideals of the politics of inclusion.

Thus, my argument here is that the dark past has functioned as an imaginary in opposition to which understandings of the present are produced (see Drinkwater, 2005:229–30). I believe that this is worth expanding on a bit further. Consider how Spivak (1999:1) warns of the dangers of placing colonialism securely in the past, thereby blinding us to how practices of our present continue to constrain and repress the subaltern. Post-institutional analysis of intellectual disability is about recognising the parallel with disability politics: consider the glum black-and-white pictures which are often used to illustrate books on the history of disability (see Grunewald, 2008, for an illustrating example), the vacuous facial expressions of the disabled, and the large institutional buildings in the background. This is a way of visualising power as 'that dark era which we have left behind', pictures that serve as mental images of what oppression looks like but which belong to history. Brown (1995:8) poignantly expresses the pitfall of this mode of analysis as a situation in which 'freedom premised upon an already vanquished enemy keeps alive, in the manner of a melancholic logic, a threat that works as domination in the form of an absorbing ghostly battle with the past'.

So, what if the ghosts we are fighting do not constitute the only, or even the primary, threat? Verstraete (2007:58) proposes that the 'modern independent-autonomous-sufficient-free subjectivity' of disability research is often considered to be the only alternative to a crushing and oppressive past. Simultaneously, questions regarding whether this view of subjectivity itself may be an expression of power are effectively precluded when walking backwards into the future, anxiously watching for the spectres of institutionalisation.

As is argued by Brown (1995:3), critical intentions are often figured within the same paradigms that had previously brought about the powers which they set out to contest. The recurring starting point of designating 'choice', 'autonomy', and 'independence' as the appropriate yardsticks of disability services effectively overlooks how these ideals, taken on their own, compose a mode of putting subjects into being. In this vein, Verstraete (2007:60) argues that an 'accent on autonomy, self-sufficiency and independence [. . .] tends to confirm who we are at this very moment rather than questioning this kind of subjectivity' (see also Jordan, 2010). Similarly, Clifford Simplican (2015:65) states that disability scholarship which advocates 'emancipation' often hinges its analysis on liberal models of agency, and therefore it is often projected that the first step of successful disability activism is to convincingly argue that disabled people are capable of 'independence' and 'self-determination' as understood within this tradition. At the same time, the possibility that these ideals, by themselves, may be vehicles and tools of power is ignored.

In other words, my argument here is that the frequent insistence of disability scholarship and advocates to propagate for 'citizenship' and 'independence' often does not sufficiently address its own ideological underpinnings (see Brown, 2008:113). Although more or less all research on intellectual disability is very critical of state power, in its lyricism of the cold monster, it fails to detect government when it is no longer cold and monstrous but increasingly dispersed and embedded in promises of freedom.

Post-structuralism and intellectual disability

In light of this, there is a need to address disability without taking its pre-political existence for granted and without viewing 'citizenship' and 'inclusion' as being equal to 'emancipation'. Within disability studies, a number of significant efforts have contributed to such a theoretical perspective.

First, knowledge of brains and bodies is intimately linked to the organisation of political communities, as Malabou (2008:55) states: 'any vision of the brain is necessarily political'. In this context, this suggests that the brain is a projection surface for ideas about who is worthy of inclusion, indeed, that the brain is a place where the power intrinsic to separate 'normal' from 'pathological' is expressed. The relationships among biology, normalcy, and power have been a main concern of the growing body of literature branded as 'Crip theory'. By putting queer theorisations of sex and sexuality into dialogue with disability, 'Crip' can be seen as an umbrella term for a number of theoretical attempts to understand how disability is socially constituted and responded to. This perspective is most clearly connected to the work of Robert McRuer (2006), who branded the term, but scholars such as Rosemarie Garland Thomson (1997, 2012), Dan Goodley (2014), and Lennard Davis (1995, 2002), among others, share many of its important characteristics. Often focusing on the construction of the 'normal' body, or the 'normate' as Garland Thomson (1997) denotes the idea of a human being who functions fully at all times, Crip theorisations of disability help us recognise how disability is normatively imbued and always related to an implicit ideal of 'able' functioning. Viewed this way, thus, there is no disability prior to the yardstick that decides which bodies qualify as 'able'.

Now, all of these theorists avoid presuming the natural and pre-political status of disability and the unequivocally liberating force of citizenship. Instead, disability, power, and subjectivity are understood as tightly nestled together through an array of governmental practices and systems of knowledge. Starting from the work of Foucault and Butler, I will also analyse 'intellectual disability' as inseparable from power and normativity. Therefore, some of the theoretical propositions of these two and a few other philosophers are what we turn to next.

Inclusion/exclusion

The politics of post-institutionalisation is structured by the terminology of inside and outside societal belonging, where independence, participation, and integration are denominators of 'inclusion'. The first theoretical theme I want to address concerns how we should understand this way of making sense of politics.

Inside/outside as a model for understanding social organisation relies on a spatial metaphor, implying a sphere of inclusion and an outside space of exclusion. Daly (2006:3) argues that, by the introduction of this metaphor, the dominant way of figuring social injustice has shifted during the last decades, from the perception that inequality is the main problem, hierarchical in nature, to the view of a perceived rift between those who are 'included' and those who are 'excluded', most often in relation to the sphere of 'full citizenship'. Thus, our imaginary of injustice has turned horizontal. Provided this imaginary, the most prominent feature of calls for 'inclusion' is that they presuppose the existence of a border separating 'included' from 'excluded' without questioning the existence of the border as such. This is a conceptual feature of this lexicon and an ontology underpinning its use. In effect, this means that 'inclusion' and 'exclusion' appear as mutually constitutive opposites (see Daly, 2006:10).

However, following Derrida's analysis of language as a system of perpetually deferred differences (see Derrida, 2001), this binary cannot be relied upon as a stable referent of the realities it seeks to name; the division between inside and outside is always threatened with displacement, implosion, and suspension (see Morton, 2003:26). Attempts to uphold the separation between inside and outside can therefore be analysed as ways of consolidating how we understand social order and the efforts to enclose otherness within the sphere of exclusion as a protection of our sense of community. As I will return to later on, this is why it has been so important to separate intellectual disability from normalcy and to anchor it in a biology of deviancy; it is a way of safeguarding a notion of subjectivity founded on ideals of reason and rationality. Still, as Butler notes, any such separation will mean that the normativity of inclusion incorporates the outside as its condition of possibility. Clearly influenced by Derrida, she describes this as a latent presence of what is excluded in the form of a threat of a terrifying return (Butler, 1993:26–7); constitutive outsides are composed of exclusions that are internal to the system as its own 'non-thematizeable necessity', emerging as incoherence, disruptions, and threats to social order (Butler, 1993:13). Whatever norm of appropriate and normal functioning that goes into our senses of 'inclusion' is perpetually haunted by what it has excluded in order to appear to be a reasonable characterisation of humanity.

In this way, 'inclusion' denotes a particular kind of movement, and citizenship has become a standard term for how this movement is substantiated. It follows that the ultimate goal of 'citizenship inclusion' cannot be a world without borders that separate insiders from outsiders (see Thomassen, 2005); it can merely be a world in which inclusion and exclusion, by means of citizenship, are allocated differently. This suggests that there is a latent danger that demands for inclusion re-inscribe what is seen as its content and prerequisites. In a sense, this was my criticism of some tendencies within social scientific intellectual disability research earlier: by parsing political demands in the terminology of 'citizenship inclusion', the subjectivity presumed as necessary for being included is being reprised. The same problem is highlighted in Homi Bhabha's (2005:xiii) discussion on the logic of post-colonial integration, which he describes as 'normalizing discourses of progress and civility [. . .] that only 'tolerate' differences they are able to culturally assimilate into their own *singular* terms, or appropriate within their own *untranslated* traditions' [italics in original quote].

Furthermore, discourses of 'citizenship' and 'inclusion' direct our focus towards questions of *entry* and *exit* at the expanse of how the normativity of citizenship operates *within* spheres of inclusion (see Daly, 2006:4). Bhabha continues by stating that his example of a racial optic can serve as a stand-in for any form of social difference or discrimination. For him, the limits of inclusion follows the ability of certain Others to meet citizenship requirements of civility and lawful participation. As Isin (2009:372) notes, citizenship always means more than being an insider; it also means mastering conducts that are seen as necessary to be a full member of society. In other words, 'inclusion' requires subjects seen as worthy of inclusion. Not only is there the power to exclude but also the power to formulate and transpire the goals that the excluded strive for and the ideals they must meet in order to be seen as worthy of inclusion.

Subjectivity

It follows from what has been said so far that the division between 'included' and 'excluded' operates by structuring how we perceive our world and therefore also how our identities are shaped. It is a binary that is tied to several other divisions that will reappear throughout this book, as for example between 'normal' and 'abnormal', 'healthy' and 'pathological, 'reason' and 'lack of reason', and 'independence' and 'dependence'. The formation of subjects takes place in such discursive systems of concepts organised together. I will here introduce how I see this.

When framing the problem of this book, I referred to an ideal 'citizen-subject' at some occasions, defined by reason, rationality, and independence. Much feminist and post-colonial theory has analysed the racialized and gendered nature of this ideal, and Crip theorisations of citizenship have analysed how this concept is tied to the ideal of an 'able' body (see Davis, 2002; Jordan, 2010). Bridget Anderson (2013) argues in a slightly different terminology that there is a 'liberal individual' at the heart of 'liberal citizenship', formed around the idea of self-ownership of their body, their labour, and their mind. Hence, inherent to modern political thinking is a story of an 'I' that is exercising self-mastery through reason – an idea that can be traced back to the moral philosophy and epistemology of Kant and the individualism of Descartes and which designates autonomy, competence, and reason as necessary preconditions of citizenship (see Shildrick, 2000, in Clifford Simplican, 2015:99; Erevelles, 2002:6). It is important to point out that this ideal links political and societal belonging to the inner life of the individual, precisely since we enter relations with the political community as 'citizens' by merit of our capacity to meet this model of subjectivity. I will refer to this ideal construction as 'the humanist subject', in which 'humanism', following Foucault, is understood as a set of propositions that tie us to a specific notion of personhood.

Now, the humanist subject is central to divisions between inclusion and exclusion and therefore also to how subjectivities are shaped in relation to this division. As Morton (2003:37) notes, throughout Western history, certain people, concepts, and ideas have been defined as 'other' in relation to 'civilized' society, and it is by the relegation of such Others to the exterior of normalcy that the sovereignty of the humanist subject is guaranteed. This has some important implications for how we understand people as belonging to certain identity categories. According to Butler (2005), the process of coming into being as a subject will always be framed by discourses which are prior to us but nevertheless constitute the conditions of possibility of our emergence. This means that categories such as 'abnormal' and 'normal', for example, are always already there when we appear to inhabit them. We cannot choose exactly who we want to be, as a crude reading of the humanist subject would suggest, but come into being provided a set of already-established categories. In turn, inhabiting the position of the 'citizen' – as understood within the humanist tradition – means coming into being in relation to a prior normativity which designates the capacities that 'citizenship' requires.

In this context, Butler's (1990, 1993) notion of 'performativity' provides a theoretical vocabulary to understand the way subjectivity is formed in relation to the social categories that define the kinds of people we are. It is important to note that Butler does not suggest that identity itself is performed, as in 'acted', but that performativity as a societal and ritualised repetition of norms is the condition which makes it possible for subjects to emerge. There is a grammar to how we come into being, which is prior to us and therefore gives rise to the defining lack that was central to how Lacan imagined the psyche (see Žižek, 2006:3). In Butler's (1993:xxi–xxiv) analysis, discursively constructed categorisations function by being unattainable: we can never be reassured of belonging once and for all in her analysis to the ideals of 'masculinity' and 'femininity'. But since such categories still precondition our recognition as subjects, they are necessary to our sense of identity, which means that our behaviours will iterate prior ideals of 'maleness' or 'femaleness' in order to secure our belonging. The performativity of subjects is how our behaviour unconsciously mimics the unattainable ideals of subject-positions to produce our identity. Along the same lines, McRuer (2006) argues that 'ability' is a ritualised repetition of norms, operating through 'compulsory able-bodiedness' as an unattainable ideal. In the concluding pages of Chapter 2, I will discuss how the ritualised repetition of norms can be understood with respect to intellectual disability.

By recognising these things, we are able to put forth a number of crucial questions regarding intellectual disability: Why are these people understood as belonging to the same category? What do they have in common? What forces are deciding on the line of demarcation which allows for their existence? How are they constituted as citizen-subjects, and what happens if they fail to meet the implicit norms that characterise members of the citizenry? In response to such questions, we shall now turn to discuss 'government' and 'biopolitics'.

Biopolitical government

The overarching analytical term of my examination is 'biopolitics', in a sense functioning as an umbrella under which the earlier discussions on inclusion/exclusion and subjectivity are incorporated in the context of this book. This does not imply that this term will return as an analytical tool in every argument I develop but rather that it functions as a general description of how I see intellectual disability politics as an instance of government. The propositions presented so far all point towards a radically different understanding of government and power than the one I criticised in my discussion on social scientific research on disability a few pages back. Tremain (2005:9) argues that a 'juridico-discursive' conception of power dominates social scientific research on disability, where government is understood as centralised and power as possessed by authorities external to the subjects being repressed. To understand intellectual disability as an instance of 'biopolitics', as analysed by Foucault, is to break with this perspective.

For Foucault, biopolitics is a form of government that takes the individuals and the totality of the population as its target, emerging during the 18th century when the importance of sovereign control over territory decreased. He describes the advent of this form of rule as the orchestration of:

> the set of mechanisms through which the basic biological features of the human species became the object of a political strategy, of a general strategy of power, in other words, how, starting from the eighteenth century, modern western societies took on board the fundamental biological fact that human beings are a species.
>
> (2007:1)

The concept of 'population' is here understood as stretching from the biological rootedness of human beings to the social practices that help us navigate society, constituting a field of realities that compose the pertinent elements for mechanisms of power to act on (Foucault, 2007:75). Hence, the ways we conduct ourselves, understand ourselves, and regulate our behaviour are all targets of government as well as our material composition and the way they mix with those of others to form a populace. Foucault (2007:70) here describes that 'the population' is conceived of as a set of processes to be managed. The range of this field of management is reflected in the terminology of use: *biopolitics* (or 'biopower') *is the power of life itself*. Seeing 'intellectual disability as biopolitics' is to understand this condition as the outcome of and embedded in the government of human life.

Under the previous heading, I discussed how subjects – by 'performativity' – are shaped in processes of internalising social norms and categorisations. A central aspect of that regards how subject formation takes shape provided socially mediated conceptions, ideas, and presumed assumptions, concerning what it means to be human. The link between subjectivity and government highlights a specific role of normativity in Foucault's analysis. The emergence of biopolitics meant a growing importance of the norm, since a power whose objective is life itself needs continuous regulatory and corrective mechanisms. Such a power cannot display itself in its 'murderous splendour', as he dramatically formulates it (Foucault, 1990:144). It rather works by distributions around the norm in processes that are largely driven by self-regulating individuals. In order to be a full member of society, one has to achieve 'normality' through working on oneself (see Davis, 2002:106).

In a considerably broader sense than dictated by its everyday use, Foucault sees ideas about normalcy – produced and upheld through science, culture, media, folklore, and so on – as examples of 'knowledge'. In the spirit of Nietzsche, this means that questions of knowledge do not pertain to the distinction between 'false' and 'true' but are questions of truth themselves – of how 'truths' are *made* and internalised into our worldviews (see Simons, 1995:19). In Foucault's analysis of government, power and knowledge are always intertwined, where knowledge is attributed with the power to produce subjects and where power works by deciding what qualifies as knowledge. Of special importance here, as Urla and Terry (1995) among others have argued, is the production of scientific knowledge functioning as an instrument for making the population governable; by segmenting it, ascribing to it specific characteristics, and mapping its behaviour at an increasing level of detail (see Foucault, 2007:77–9; Rose, 2006). Concurrently, biopolitics also implies management on the micro level, targeting the individual and their behaviour, where each human being represents an unfulfilled promise of improvement. Foucault (see 1990:139–42) continuously engages this dual nature of government, exercised on the individual body and mind and on the population as a whole.

Now, an important implication of this understanding of power is that we have to abandon the view that there is a dichotomous relationship between subjects acting freely and the government intervening in such processes of self-creation. Government does not have to rely on repressing and constraining freedom but can also work by putting in place a specific configuration of freedom and shaping the fields of action where it is exercised, meaning that it is, *acting on* rather than *suppressing* individual agency. It follows that the government of the population does not always require force and coercion but may just as well function through self-regulation and internalisation of certain norms, that is, by moulding the capacity of individuals to govern themselves (see Cruikshank, 1999; Rose, 1999), which is why Foucault calls government 'the conduct of conduct' (Foucault, 2000:341; see also 1982:789 for an alternative translation). For example, in Chapter 5 I will elaborate on how group homes for people with intellectual disabilities are not only places where freedom is restricted but also where individuals are shaped to understand themselves as 'free' in a certain sense and are impelled to exercise this freedom in specific ways. Furthermore, rather than an inherently bad thing that should be discarded, power should instead be seen as a necessity and inevitable feature of social organisation. Thus, to point out that a certain practice, for example of classifying 'intellectual disability', is an instance of power does not imply that it should be abandoned.

However, in order to have an informed discussion revolving around such practices, we need to acknowledge their social and political nature.

Final remarks

As evidenced by the chapter outline and theoretical discussion above, I will engage with a broad range of issues and topics that speaks of intellectual disability politics. Rather than a systematised selection of well-defined materials or anything of the sort, the theoretical arguments will be the glue that holds the subsequent chapters together. It follows that the general method of this book will be to discuss a set of concepts and ideas, such as 'inclusion', 'normality', 'intellectual disability', and 'citizenship', by theoretical analysis of a variety of empirical sources. For example, the material will consist of historical and contemporary policy texts, scientific works, and philosophical arguments, but also of, all in all, 40 interviews with support workers, bureaucrats, and disability activists and advocates. The materials will be presented further as they appear throughout the book.

I want to wrap up this introductory chapter by offering up a few notes concerning the ethical considerations that have gone into this work. First, it should be noted that this book stems from my background working within disability services, as a street-level support worker, then for a brief period as a bureaucrat and evaluator. Along the way, I have come to know many people labelled as 'intellectually disabled'. These experiences have caused a great sense of personal distress revolving around the border which separated me from the people with intellectual disabilities that I met. What does it mean to provide support for these people? What makes my outlook on things appear to be more valuable than theirs in most contexts? How are we controlling members of this group, and how am I complicit? In a sense, this book is an attempt to find a language to make sense of these experiences.

Second, a central ethical stance is conspicuous in the theoretical perspective: my primary interest is not how people with intellectual disabilities view the world, what is in their best interest, or how they function, but how the condition is constructed and governed. Indeed, it appears to me that projects that seek to represent intellectual disability or the interests of individuals labelled as such not only have a tendency to slate over considerable differences within the group but also assign themselves the role of speaking *for* people with this condition in a way that rests on an implicit and problematic hierarchy. In light of the historical treatment of people with intellectual disabilities, I believe that it is imperative that disability research does not make itself complicit in that. Rather, the point for me is to create spaces for politicisation, spaces from which people with intellectual disabilities can speak, and to do this by uprooting presumed assumptions about the inherent deficiencies of the group's members.

Last, for the interviews with political activists with intellectual disability, I have been granted ethical approval by the Swedish Board of Research Ethics, which, in turn, requires that I refrain from using their real names.

2 Pathology

This chapter focuses on how 'intellectual disability' is constituted as an object of knowledge for government purposes, that is, how questions concerning what this condition is are answered by medical, para-medical, and psychological science and how the answers provided are integral to the government of the group. This will serve as a necessary background to understand the politics of post-institutionalisation, which is underpinned by a classificatory and medical conception of intellectual disability.

The chapter proceeds in three analytical steps. I will start with a discussion of the history and present of classification and diagnosis, arguing that 'intellectual disability' is a biopolitical construction that dresses up normative judgements of deviancy as scientific facts. Thereafter, I will go on to discuss how medical depictions of intellectual disability returns deviancy to the body, thereby masking the inherent politics of the diagnosis. To conclude the chapter, I will discuss what these arguments imply for our conception of disability and argue for an understanding that bridges the divide between politics and nature.

Classification

To start with: intellectual disability is popularly understood as a condition of deficient cognitive functioning, which, in turn, has extensive effects on the living conditions of the individuals labelled so (Bennett, 2006:341–5; Harris, 2006:3–5; Carr & O'Reilly, 2007a:17–27). By this view, the objective of disability politics is related to the social arrangements affecting the lives of those diagnosed, as through, for example, care organisation, group home living, and sheltered employment, whilst the condition as such is rendered outside the scope of politics. As I will elaborate upon in the following, this way of making sense of the relationship between diagnosis and politics neglects how governmental concerns, from the outset, have been integrated into classificatory practices. Thus, rather than a biological condition that politics answer to, I will argue that intellectual disability is a political construction that classification seeks to dress up as a neutral and natural fact about certain people.

It shall be noted that this is far from the first account seeking to lay bare the social and political dimensions of how intellectual disability is defined by

22 *Introduction*

analysing the history of measurement technologies and definitions (see Rapley, 2004; McClimens, 2007; Carlson, 2010; Sleeter, 2010; Goodey, 2011; Simpson, 2012; Altermark, 2015). The first part of this chapter, focusing on classification, should be read as an addition to this literature, where I analyse how historical continuities and discontinuities in definitions impose limits concerning what becomes possible to think and know about the group (see Carlson, 2010:17). However, the account presented here differs from the cited works by using Foucault's biopolitics to discuss the relationship between knowledge and government, which in the subsequent chapters will prove necessary to make sense of post-institutionalisation and the politics of citizenship inclusion.

Presently, all globally used classification systems (the American Association of Intellectual and Developmental Disabilities [AAIDD], the fifth Diagnostic and Statistical Manual of Mental Disorders [DSM-5], and the tenth version of the International Classification of Diseases [ICD-10]) define intellectual disability as the concurrent featuring of intellectual and adaptive behaviour deficits that can be scientifically measured and which appear during the developmental period of life. Although classificatory systems have undergone repeated revisions, the coupling of psychometrically deficient intelligence and behavioural problems is still the foundation of how intellectual disability is understood. This understanding of the condition implies that there is no single cause or prognosis pertaining to all diagnosed individuals. Thus, 'intellectual disability' covers inherited syndromes, traumatic injuries, and more than 1,000 genetic conditions that have been associated with the condition (Tartaglia et al., 2007:98). Still, in a majority of people diagnosed, there are no known biological explanations (Bennett, 2006:343; McDermott et al., 2007:9).[1] Moreover, it is maintained that genetic, medical, psychological, and environmental factors all contribute to determine the level of cognitive impairment (Bennett, 2006:343), that many malfunctions can conjoin in one individual, and, furthermore, that cognitive limitations are often added to by perceptual and motor impairments (Harris, 2006:12; McDermott et al., 2007:3).

Despite the heterogeneity of sub-diagnoses and differences as concerns functioning and service needs contained within the category of 'intellectual disability', it is important to note that the condition is seen as a specific way to be in the world. Understanding how this makes sense – political sense – is to start to understand intellectual disability as an expression of biopolitics.

Psychometric histories of our present

First, as Goodey (2011:1) notes, the idea that 'intelligence' is a defining characteristic of humanity is distinctively modern, combining a strong belief in the capacity of science to make the world measureable with the hallmarks of modern philosophical conceptions of humans as mastering the world by reason. The introduction of intelligence testing during the early 20th century considerably changed understandings of mental deficits (Goodey, 2011:1). These changes involved making possible a clear-cut distinction between physical and mental impairments, which had previously been blurred, and differentiating mental deficits from mental illnesses (Goodey & Stainton, 2001:225; Carlson, 2010:24). Furthermore, psychometrics introduced scientific rigour as an overriding ideal. As is suggested by Jenkins (1999:17 in Rapley, 2004:32), throughout the 20th century the statistical plotting of normal-curve distributed intelligence has been a primary tool of defining intellectual deficiency. An important reason for its success was the appearance that IQ presented accurate and objective representations of naturally existing phenomena. Hence, the dawn of IQ testing exemplifies what Canguilhem (1991:47–8) analyses as a shift from a qualitative to a quantitative conception of sickness and abnormality, where pathological phenomena went from being seen as differences of sorts to measureable variations which could be plotted around a statistical norm (see Vailly, 2008:2532).

Thus, from the outset, the notion of 'intelligence' has been at the heart of diagnosis. The dominating conception of today can be exemplified by Harris's (2006:99) statement that 'intellect' refers to 'the power of thought', distinguishable from perceptions and emotions. This is congruent with Jensen's (1998:336 in Rapley, 2004:36) description of intellectual disability as a 'thinking disability'. Intelligence is understood as the capability of understanding and solving problems (Harris, 2006:99) or, as stated by the AAIDD (2010:15) clinical guidebook,

> *Intelligence* is a general mental ability. It includes reasoning, planning, solving problems, thinking abstractly, comprehending complex ideas, learning quickly, and learning from experience. . . . As reflected in this definition, intelligence is not merely book learning, a narrow academic skill, or test-taking smarts. Rather, it reflects a broader and deeper capacity for comprehending our surroundings – catching on, making sense of things, or figuring out what to do.

This way of comprehending 'intelligence' rose to prominence during the first decades of the 20th century. From the 1820s onwards, Western states had begun to amass statistics on various forms of human deviancy (Hacking, 1986:161). Over the course of the second half of the 19th century, there was an explosion of interest in deviancies of the intellect. During the second half of the 19th century, intellect was widely referred to as the capacity to 'adjust' to different situations and to do so by means of 'reason' (see Axelsson, 2007:223). The idea has a clear origin in Enlightenment conceptions of humans as defined by reason, which, for example, can be seen in how Paton (1905:29) argued that the adult human mind is characterised by the ability to rise above sensations and emotions to produce detached thinking governed by rationality. Here, Paton echoes Kant's self-governing subject, capable of taming their emotions by laws of reason, an idea that had a significant impact on a number of early thinkers on 'normal' and 'deficient' intelligence (see Goodey, 2011:210).

Another prominent figure of Enlightenment thinking who influenced early conceptions of intelligence was John Locke, whose notion of a strictly intellectual disability, differentiated from insanity and lunacy, recurs in the literature at the time (see Brady, 1865:6; Harris, 2006:140; Goodey, 2011:12, 246). Consequently, the growing concerns of 'mental deficiency' around the turn of the century came to echo Locke's philosophical efforts to differentiate 'normal' humans, characterised by faculties of reason, and groups (such as 'changelings' and 'idiots') that lacked this characteristic (Locke's arguments will be thoroughly dealt with in Chapter 3; see Goodey, 2011:313–15; Clifford Simplican, 2015:22). In his thorough account of early classification, Goodey argues that Locke's conception of human beings as defined by reason was central to how 'deficient intelligence' emerged as a scientific object of inquiry. Hence, prior to the breakthrough of psychometrics and its figuration of intelligence as a measureable quantity was a general idea of the 'normal' and rational human mind; it was a notion of intelligence moulded after the ideals of Enlightenment humanism. Provided the stronghold of this conception, any deficiencies became noticeable and perceived as troublesome, which is aptly captured by Clouston (1883:2):

> The whole conduct of things in the world is necessarily so based on the assumption that every man is a responsible being with a sound mind, that any exception to this, when it occurs, has a very startling effect.

This notion of what defines humans was, of course, pivotal to perceptions of the relationship between the individual and the state, that is, to the idea of 'the citizen'. The well-ordered society needed a citizenry composed of self-restrained and autonomous individuals guided by reason, as Herbert Spencer (1890 in Axelsson, 2007:48) – one of the inventors of psychometrics – argued. As a result, an important objective of the state became the targeting of individuals seen as unable to meet the overarching ideals of a self-ruling citizenry (see Axelsson, 2007). For people perceived as lacking proper faculties of reason, 'intelligence' was used to form judgements concerning their ability to fulfil civic responsibilities, seen in how Tredgold (1908:2 in Rapley, 2004:60) defined 'mental deficiency' as a state of 'incomplete cerebral development' with the result that 'the person affected is unable to perform his duties as a member of society in the position of life to which he is born'. 'Intelligence' thus functioned as something more than a description of an individual characteristic; it was also a normative yardstick linked to ideals of citizenship and the defining characteristics of humanity; the linkages between a philosophical ideal subject, citizenship, and scientific conceptions of intelligence together came to facilitate the envisioning of the 'mentally deficient' person as an alien and abject outsider.

In parallel to the emergence of the conception of 'intelligence', the first decades of the 20th century saw the linking together of numerous societal problems and people perceived as having deficient intelligence. In their preface to the popular summary of the Royal Commission of the Care and Control of the Feebleminded (preceding the UK Mental Deficiency Act of 1913), Darwin et al. (1909) stated that people of this group were 'unhappy in themselves, a sorrow and burden to their families, and a growing source of expense and danger to the community'. In a similar way, Henderson (1901:180–1) proposed that 'the evils of feeblemindedness' constituted a 'perpetual source of danger and injury' in society.

In this way, poverty, criminality, and social unrest could all be understood in light of mental degradation and defective intelligence (see Henderson, 1901; Webb & Webb, 1912; Davey, 1914; Kelynack, 1915) and, by that, managing the 'mentally deficient' became a question of ensuring the social order (see Binet & Simon, 1914:10). A special problem concerned people of 'deficient intelligence' who could easily pass as 'normal', not bearing any visible or physical characteristics, which meant that they risked going undetected (Binet & Simon, 1914:vi; Galton, 1914 in Penrose, 1954:11). Henderson (1901) argued that such individuals of a 'feeble and distorted nature' were bent towards anti-social conduct (252), that they were particularly pliable to temptation and distress (252), and that when persons of this group were surrounded by a vicious environment, they were inclined to develop a craving for stimulants, arousing 'the beast within' (253).

In this way, 'intelligence' facilitated a linking together of certain social anxieties with a specific group of individuals seen as lacking human reason (see Walmsley, 2005:51). At the same time, ideas concerning the hereditary nature of mental deficits and the increasing biologisation of how the mind was interpreted put the quality of the population at stake, leading Darwin et al. (1909) to declare that the procreation of such people 'threatens the race with progressive deterioration'. Eugenics would emerge as the most obvious expression of how concerns of the quality of the citizenry and the hereditary nature of deficient intelligence were linked together, as is expressed by Kelynack (1915:vi–vii):

> The nation is awake to the urgent necessity for securing the conservation of its children. Every form of defectiveness must be reduced to its minimum, and all varieties of preventible [sic] disorder must be dealt with by effective agencies, if we are to provide healthy citizens for coming days.

Provided these sentiments, and at roughly the same time, the countries in Northern Europe and America created laws and policies aiming to separate, educate, and prevent from mating the mentally deficient (see Stiker, 1999:127–30, 155–6; Walmsley, 2005:52; Grunewald, 2008:68–73, 107–9). These laws were closely connected to psychiatric and psychological accounts of the time, wherein the scientific description of deficiency and the urgency of intervention appeared to be intertwined (see Henderson, 1901). Davey's introduction and commentary to the UK Mental Deficiency Act is illuminating in this respect:

> Of the gravity of the present state of things, there is no doubt. The mass of facts that we have collected, the statements of our witnesses, and our own personal visits and investigations compel the conclusion that there are numbers of mentally defective persons whose training is neglected, over whom no sufficient control is exercised, and whose wayward and irresponsible lives are productive of crime and misery, of much injury and mischief to themselves and others, and of much continuous expenditure wasteful to the community and to individual families.
>
> (Davey, 1914:2)

However, this gave rise to a new problem, namely how members of this group were to be segmented:

> Our third principle is that if the mentally defective are to be properly considered and protected as such, it is necessary to ascertain who they are and where they are, and to bring them into relation with the local authority. This should, we think, be done chiefly through the agency of the education authority and other public or *quasi*-public authorities without any undue invasion of the privacy of the family.
>
> (in Davey, 1914:6, italics in original)

This aptly captures Foucault's proposition of biopolitics: in order to govern the population, the population needs to be known. And it was provided this background that IQ testing and psychometrics rose to prominence (see Axelsson, 2007:58; Hansson, 2007:63; Carlson, 2010:47).

The French psychologist Alfred Binet invented the first IQ test to help the Parisian school board decide which children needed special schooling (Borkowski et al., 2007:262; Kring et al., 2007:84). The method quickly spread throughout Europe and over the Atlantic. Previously, estimating cognitive capabilities had been a difficult and time consuming process, complicated by the fact that some people were considered 'mentally deficient' without any visible or physical characteristics. Psychometrics provided a fitting response to these problems, conceptualising intelligence as an invisible characteristic, residing *within* rather than on the surface of the individual. Thus, IQ testing arrived with the promise of solving the problem of the group falling precisely below the 'normal range' whose appearance did not reveal obvious signs of malfunction. Terman (1916), who would translate and adopt the Binet-Simon test for American conditions (still known as the Stanford-Binet test), described the potential benefits:

> It is safe to presume that within the reasonably near future intelligence tests will bring tens of thousands of these high grade cases under surveillance and protection of society. This will ultimately result in curtailing the reproduction of feeblemindedness and in the elimination of a vast amount of crime, pauperism and industrial inefficiency.

In this way, the interconnectedness of societal normativity, state institutions, governmental concerns, and scientific knowledge came to constitute a central instance of biopolitics. As is explicitly indicated by several of the early thinkers of cognitive impairment who have been quoted here, absolutely central to this was the interlinking of conceptions of normalcy and cognitive deficiency (see also Henderson, 1901; Mercier, 1905):

> The preceding description of "Mind" will apply to Minds of all kinds. It is therefore necessary to investigate the characteristics special to the feeble mind

and this can only be done by erecting a standard of the normal mind for purposes of comparison.

(Sherlock, 1911:70)

Since every community consists of individuals varying very greatly in the
extent of their mental development, it is necessary to explain what is meant
by 'normal', and to state what is the criterion adopted to differentiate the
normal from the mentally defective.

(Tredgold et al., 1912:66)

Hence, the construction of the 'normal' mind was imperative for the differentiation
of the 'feeble' mind. In this way, psychometrics exemplifies a way of *constituting*
what it presents itself as, *describing* by reference to a prior norm of how human
beings *should* function. To speak with Butler (1993:xiii), this exemplifies the
constitutive force of normativity, where an ideal of human reason simultaneously
institutes an outside threat which must be known and controlled.

In summary, the importance of psychometrics during the first decades of the
20th century can be explained by its capacity to pinpoint individuals already seen
as problematic and as requiring governmental management; it was a tool of rule
as much as a tool of science. By psychometric knowledge, IQ was linked to how
citizens understood their rights and duties and thereby became instrumental to
a functioning public (Zenderland, 2001 in Axelsson, 2007:60), at the same time
both an expression and a reinforcement of societal norms concerning which
capacities characterise humanity. 'Mental deficiency' emerged as a name for
those that failed to be proper citizens. As Clifford Simplican (2015:22, 50) notes,
the philosophical construction of a subject of deliberation and self-management
was incorporated by early psychology and psychiatry in order to lend credence
to their scientific mapping of deviancy, which, on the other hand, provided tools
that could be used to organise government interventions. And in this way, I argue,
the classification of intellectual disability came to embody the normativity of the
humanist subject.

Classification today

Of course, the foregoing is not mere history but historicity as a method of denatural-
ising present knowledge. From our current historical location, we can easily recognise the normative investments made in historical ways of naming and speaking of
intellectual disability, but we are less inclined to see how the history of intelligence
testing is inscribed into contemporary understandings of the condition.

Through the shifts in classificatory criteria, lay conceptions, and psychological
theorisations, what has remained constant to the notion of 'intelligence' is the fact
that it has been the outcome of a historically contingent social consensus concerning
what is 'normal' and what is 'abnormal', as Goodey (2011:1) expresses it. Thus, the
mutually constitutive relationship between 'norm' and 'deviancy' is a discursive

feature which also permeates present conceptions of intellectual disability: just like before, today's clinical depictions often define intellectual disability by comparing it to the development of 'normal' individuals (Carr & O'Reilly, 2007b:71). This normalcy, furthermore, seems to be moulded after very similar ideas of adaptability and self-regulation which were integral to the first modern conceptions of intelligence. Note, for example, how Borkowski et al. (2007:271–3) proposes that the defining characteristic of people in this group is their lack of 'self-regulation', denoting processes of monitoring one's own learning and development, and being able to consciously oversee and control one's behaviour. In a similar way, Carr & O'Reilly (2007b:74) refer to an intellectually disabled 'personality profile' which is characterised by a lack of motivation to learn new skills due to a lack of self-control. There is an important linkage here to the idea of 'adaptability' as conceived of in 19th century conceptions of 'intelligence' and further back to the philosophical notions of a subject of reason; being able to conform to various social situations, to manage one's behaviour, and thus to fulfil one's duties is central to being a citizen.

How does this relate to the classificatory practices of today? First, it shall be noted that IQ is not and never has been a straightforward measurement of intelligence, but of each individual's intelligence *compared to the rest of the population*. IQ scales are normed and tests constructed so that the average member of the population (that the specific test is constructed for) has an IQ of 100 (Hacking, 2007:316). This follows the outline of Galton's groundbreaking application of normal distribution to individual psychological features, with the consequence that IQ tests do not measure intelligence in absolute terms but in relation to a statistical norm. Following Jenkins (1999:17 in Rapley, 2004:32), this suggests that 'intellectual disability' could not have existed before the invention of normal distribution.

Now, placing the cutoff point at an IQ of 70 designates two standard deviations below average, which means that 2.27% of any population assumed falls under the bar if the test is correctly constructed and intelligence is normally distributed. Following these assumptions, the 2.27% of any population performing worst on tests will meet the IQ criterion for intellectual disability. Consequently, this placement of the cutoff precludes the possibility that more than about 1 to 3% of the population is intellectually disabled (see Carr & O'Reilly, 2007a:29). This means that there are no necessary linkages between IQ testing and the biology of cognitive functioning, precisely because IQ is a statistical measurement that only makes sense relative to the population that the test is constructed for. Already the inventors of the first IQ test, Binet and Simon (in Carlson, 2010:49), noted this:

> Our purpose is to be able to measure the intellectual capacity of a child who is brought to us in order to know whether he is normal or retarded. We should therefore, study his condition at the time and that only. We have nothing to do either with his past history or with his future; consequently we shall neglect his etiology.

Of course, as we will get back to, this seemingly contradicts the view that intellectual disability can be localised in the biophysical properties of the brain.

However, IQ testing soon became inextricably bound to hereditary explanations of 'feeblemindedness' despite the intentions of Binet and Simon (Carlson, 2010:49).

The lack of pathogens appearing precisely at an IQ of 70 begs the question why the cutoff should be placed at this particular point. In retrospect, this placement has been interpreted as stemming from a general impression that 2 to 3% of the population are intellectually disabled judging from their 'real world behaviour' (O'Reilly & Carr, 2007:126), which is to say that it is based on a judgement of what kind of behaviour passes as acceptable. Interestingly, the originator of the IQ 70 cutoff point, the psychologist David Wechsler, provided no references or guidance to any clinical studies justifying why he chose the IQ 70 yardstick when it first emerged in a 1944 article (quoted in Flynn & Widaman, 2008). In his treatment on the nature of intellectual disability, he oscillates between regarding mental deficits as quantitative and qualitative in nature. Like 'genius', he states, cognitive deficiencies are a question of difference in degree (Wechsler, 1952:133). However, as mental capacity falls below certain thresholds, it will result in behaviours that appear to be qualitatively different. The following quote follows this template:

> they actually 'look' and 'act' differently. And these differences in 'looks' and 'behaviour' can be explained by assuming that human intelligence when passing certain points takes on new configurations which for phenomeno-logical reasons we find it convenient to recognize as different totalities.
>
> (133–4)

Thus, the qualitative difference between intellectual disability and normalcy and the underlying rationale for the placement of the IQ cutoff point appears to be 'convenience' and the 'appearance' of a difference of sorts. To support this – from a scientific viewpoint rather suspect – argument, Wechsler states that one only needs to ask people who work with members of the group to get his view confirmed (133). As Carlson (2010:28–33) argues, the blurred boundaries between quantitative and qualitative differences that we can witness here have character-ised intellectual disability from the outset, for example, seen in how we measure intelligence quantitatively today, but maintain that people with this condition can be qualitatively distinguished on merits of biological causes. Justifications of the placement of the cutoff point are notably scarce in the contemporary clinical lit-erature, as well (see Bennett, 2006:343; Harris, 2006; O'Reilly & Carr, 2007). What this placement really exposes, however, is how judgement of behaviour is at the core of scientifically dressed-up justifications. Before the designation of the cutoff point, and given the lack of identifiable pathogens appearing precisely here, a prior recognition concerning who needs to be targeted must be made; it must be recognised that some people behave in ways that constitute 'pathology' and that psychometric tests are capable of doing the sorting of them. Hence, IQ tests did not provide new knowledge of a group already in existence; they invented a group which conformed to specific understandings of the relationships among intelligence, behaviour, and social problems.

At times, the clinical literature mentions that 'intellectual disability' is an 'administrative category' (see Parmeter, 2004:13–14; Borkowski et al., 2007:273; Stoneman, 2007:37), constructed in order to, for example, allow communication about the group, to direct research, and to decide eligibility for services and benefits. What these admissions actually expose are the governmental rationalities that are ingrained in understandings of intellectual disability. If we assume that intellectual disability is a natural phenomenon which exists irrespective of its measurement, the IQ criterion appears to be peculiar, verging on nonsensical. As soon as we approach IQ as a tool of biopolitics, however, these peculiarities disappear. From such a perspective, the perception that approximately 2 to 3% of the population behave in ways that call for socio-political measures is a perfectly logical starting point for psychometric measurement technologies. This may not reflect whatever intentions the inventors of intelligence testing had or the stated objectives of those upholding the practice today, but it surely reflects the inner logic of psychometrics and why certain institutions preoccupied with dividing up the population are lured in by the technology.

Today, along with psychometric testing, a diagnosis of 'intellectual disability' also requires the presence of behavioural problems. The adaptive behaviour criterion was first included in classification in 1959 by the American Association of Mental Retardation (AAMR, today AAIDD; Parmeter, 2004:10, 14) and became a feature of all classification systems during the latter half of the 20th century (McDermott, 2007:5). In the mid-20th century, there were concerns that the sole reliance on IQ testing produced a measurement that was too narrow of deficient intelligence. The introduction of adaptive behaviour was founded on the rationale that the day-to-day functioning of the individual needed to be integrated into classificatory practices. Not surprisingly, considering the entanglement of knowledge production and government, the first adaptive behaviour tests were developed to pinpoint individual characteristics of people who were already known to be intellectually disabled; the conception of adaptive behaviour was thus moulded from the group that it subsequently has been used to detect (Borthwick-Duffy, 2007:287).

Importantly, invoked into conceptions of 'adaptive behaviour' is the specification that it should be measured with reference to expectations on one's age and cultural group (ICD-10; AAIDD, 2010:16). This relative component is a basic building block of how the term is made sense of (Schalock, 2004:369, 379; Borthwick-Duffy, 2007:284). Consequently, the criterion resorts to a notion of what is considered deviant; the comparison with one's peers, from which one could expect similar adaptive skills, essentially means that it amounts to 'not as good at coping with situations of everyday life when compared with others'. In much the same way as with IQ tests, the mechanism at play is relative and designed to separate those who are deemed to be worse off than others. Furthermore, although the clinical literature on intellectual disability tends to treat 'adaptive behaviour' as separate from intelligence and analytically distant from the IQ criteria, these two components used for classifying intellectual disability have a shared history. The introduction of adaptive behaviour into classificatory schemes formalised concerns about social adjustment and appropriate behaviour which were already being heavily emphasised when mental deficiency emerged as a classificatory category (see Borthwick-Duffy, 2007:279; AAIDD, 2010:15–16).

Today, despite being a judgement on qualitative differences concerning individual behaviours, adaptive behaviour is largely measured quantitatively. Carr and O'Reilly (2007a:20–1) state that factor analysis shows adaptive behaviour falls into three categories: *conceptual skills*, which include language, literacy, numeracy skills, money skills, and self-direction; *social skills* such as the capacity to make and uphold relationships, accept responsibilities appropriate to one's age and ability level, the capacity to maintain an adequate level of self-esteem, the ability to recognise and follow informal rules for social interactions, and the ability to interpret social situations accurately; and lastly, *practical skills*, which include activities necessary for daily living such as eating, toileting, washing, dressing, meal preparation, housekeeping, mobility, and managing the occupational demands of work situations. Rather than undeniable signs of pathology, this reads as little more than a shortlist of things required to get by in contemporary Western societies. In addition, since the actual measurement of adaptive behaviour relies on information gathered through third party respondents, the core of diagnosis is qualitative judgements in which psychologists are supposed to decide whether the answers of interviewed relatives and service providers compose deficits that constitute more than two standard deviations below average (Borthwick-Duffy, 2007:286). Interpreting the result of any such judgement as indicative of an objectively existing pathology stretches the imagination, to say the least.

Hence, like IQ, adaptive behaviour appears as inapt with regards to the epistemological aspirations of the dominating understandings of intellectual disability but can be utilised as a handy instrument of biopolitics. As a complement of intelligence tests, it facilitates the creation of an overall estimation of 'personal competency' (see Schalock, 2004; Borthwick-Duffy, 2007:280), sometimes referred to as 'the essence of mental retardation [intellectual disability]' (Borthwick-Duffy, 2007:280). When considered as biopolitics, it is precisely those individuals who fail to provide for themselves, to manage their own lives, and to maintain adequacy of conduct that a system targeting deviancy would want to identify and focus suitable interventions on. As is noted by Schalock (2004:380–1), adaptive behaviour can, of course, be important for educational and other interventions, helping the individual to acquire competences to get by in present societies. Still, this does not do away with the fact that the criteria is a normatively imbued measurement of those that fail to manage life as well as their peers.

For purposes of government

The two criteria constituting 'intellectual disability' are formulated so as to pinpoint those in the general population who are worst off as concerns performances on intelligence tests and estimations of adaptive behaviour. However, nothing in these criteria indicates that 'intellectual disability' holds an ontological existence independently of how it is measured; it is there because the tests show that it is there, and the tests are motivated by the prior recognition that it is there.

The symptoms of intellectual disability are not indicative of anything else but themselves, which means that they effectively become the condition as such. This suggests that intellectual disability is a 'hypothetical construct' disguised as a 'diagnosis of disorder', as Rapley (2004:44) aptly formulates it. As a result, the symptoms of intellectual disability are equated to the label itself (see Rapley, 2004:40–3). This effectively turns into a loop of circularity as soon as one tries to render the definition of the group explanatory. Running parallel to Rapley's (2004:40–5) argument: how do we know that someone is intellectually disabled? We know this because they have sub-average intelligence according to IQ tests and because they are unable to care for themselves according to behavioural measurement assessments. Then, why do they have low IQ and why are they unable to care for themselves? It is because they are intellectually disabled, which means that they have sub-average IQ and adaptive behaviour problems. And so on. In this way the label of intellectual disability explains nothing more than the criteria constituting it. Indeed, the vocabulary of 'diagnosis', 'condition', and 'pathology', imported into psychology from medicine, appears as little more than an exercise in dressing up judgements on socially troublesome individuals in scientific and medical language.

Hence, rather than as a pre-political pathology, it seems reasonable to approach intellectual disability as a historically contingent way of making sense of individuals recognised as requiring some sort of management (see Rapley, 2004:42). This suggests that the technologies which are allegedly used to *describe* an independently existing 'disordered cognition' in fact function to *manufacture* this 'disordered cognition'. When intellectual disability first appeared, one important reason for separating this group was to be able to direct interventions so that members of the group did not procreate or create societal unrest. Today, the need to diagnose intellectual disability stems from a perception that a long-term government commitment is needed, although no longer through blatant forms of eugenics and permanent institutionalisation. Thereby, the common logic of classification is reversed: we are not dealing with a group which exists out there, detected by measurement instruments, and towards whom government is directed. Rather, we are dealing with governmental concerns, underpinning measurement instruments that are put to work to constitute subjects as 'intellectually disabled'.

For the sake of clarity, the arguments proposed here do not contest the existence of intellectual disability but are meant to engage in a discussion concerning what we take 'existence' to mean when talking about this group. Some may counter that it would be foolish to state that there are no differences between members of this group and other people, but I have merely proposed that considerations regarding *which* differences matter, of *how* and *why* they matter, and *when* they need to be acted on are all best made sense of as governmental concerns, that this has been the case throughout history and is the case today. Neither have I argued that classification is of no use: on the contrary, this diagnosis has proved highly useful in the management of the population; the problem is that this role as a tool of government is often unacknowledged and very rarely politicised. However, the use of quantitative measurement instruments to categorise differences of sorts, to designate an otherness of human reason, will inevitably produce liminal zones of ambiguity, where a firm demarcation between 'other' and 'us' is hard to maintain. The response to this problem is what we turn to next.

Return to the body

Present only by merit of their absence in the classification of intellectual disability, biological causes appear as the displaced centre of efforts to define and categorise this condition. The classificatory criteria are meant to capture pathology, but their segmenting function is relative to statistical or behavioural norms and is underpinned by ideas concerning which deviancies are judged to be troublesome. In this section, I will examine how the intellectual deficiencies detected by classification are projected onto the biology of the individual, that is, how judgements on disorder are returned to the body through psychiatric and medical knowledge. I will argue that an important ideological function of research on the medicine and biology of intellectual disability thereby is to naturalise the condition to make it appear as a biological fact rather than an outcome of government.

Histories of biological deviancy

Again, a retrospective view is needed. Over the course of the second half of the 19th century, a significant shift occurred regarding the way that 'mental deficiency' was comprehended. Previously, 'idiocy', 'imbecility', and 'feeblemindedness' had been regarded as unfortunate results of metaphysical forces – of the rage of God or the incidence of nature figured as abstraction. Thought was primarily comprehended as metaphysical in nature, sometimes linked to the divine (see Dendy, 1853:3–4 for an example). In the literature at the time, linkages between the biology of the individual and the deficient mind were rare. Concurrently, the educational efforts of Seguin and other philanthropists pictured the 'mentally deficient' as worthy targets of benevolence, and there was a widespread optimism concerning the possibilities of ameliorating the lacking intellect of such individuals (Parmeter, 2004:6). In many accounts of the group from the first half of the 19th century, it is stressed that, although people of this group cannot be figured as human in its fullest form, they deserve compassion and help.

Some 50 years later, around the turn of the century, a distinctively different view of intellectual disability had emerged. First, as I discussed earlier, 'mental deficiency' had transformed into a 'threat', linked to degeneration of the population and to various social problems. There was no longer a place for charity, pity, and optimism. Second, mental deficiency had come to be seen in ways that we recognise from today: as a medical condition to be understood by means of modern medicine. The key organ, of course, was the brain (Maudsley, 1873:40; Mercier, 1905; Paton, 1905; Mott, 1914). This perspective indicated that the study of the abnormal mind was analogous to studying any other diseased part of the body. Viewed in this way, it was possible to connect the sociology of social problems with human biology in the quest to find the causality of 'inferior indi-viduals' (Henderson, 1901:12–14). Still, as Paton (1905:230) noted in his intro-ductory textbook on psychiatry, the pathology of mental deficiencies was, to a large extent, still an enigma.

It is important to note that this shift towards a medical and biological under-standing of inferior intelligence was not primarily motivated by conclusive sci-entific findings but by new theoretical assumptions concerning how deviancy was interpreted. Very few early medical accounts have anything substantial to say about biological correlates of 'mental deficiency', but they do not hesitate to assume that such biological markers must be present, only not yet discovered. In this way, the recognition of deviancy came prior to detecting its causes. The emergence of biological explanations of intellectual disability was produced by a shift of belief system rather than of scientific discoveries; only after deviancy was recognised did psychiatry set out to search for the causes of 'mental deficiency' in the materiality of the brain.

The linkages between deficient morality, social problems, and deficient intel-ligence that I discussed earlier were also present in medical and psychiatric treat-ments of mental deficiency, as can be exemplified by Kraepelin's (1906:329) ideas about lacking intellect:

> imbeciles are naturally unable to satisfy the more difficult demands of life. Sexual relations in the present case, and in others alcohol, bad example, or a propensity to idleness, are the reefs on which they are wrecked in conse-quence of their inadequate equipment for the battle of life.

At the time, the deficits in question were, to a large extent, interpreted as heredi-tary, a view exemplified by Goddard's influential account of the Kallikak family. During the decades around the turn of the 20th century, the optimism and concern for the mentally deficient were replaced by biological determinism and a glum view of 'mental deficiency' as a motor of social unrest and degeneration. First, this made it possible to design specific measures to target people with mental deficits, separating them from the insane and the generally poor. Secondly, as the hereditary stock of society was on the line, there was an urgent need to do some-thing. And so prevention of 'mental deficiency' became a primary motivation of research as well as of policies targeting the group, driven by the eugenics move-ment and disseminated throughout the Western world.

What 'aetiology' does

One of most the important ideas which emerged during the latter half of the 19th century concerns the causation of deficient intelligence. Finding the causes of the condition has been a goal of researchers since the late 19th century and an explicit policy goal in the US, for example, since the 1960s (McDermott et al., 2007:4). What developed during the first decades of the 20th century was an ideology of origin, essentially formed around the seemingly trivial proposition that medical conditions are caused by something. As we shall turn to discuss in what follows, this simple idea has played a significant role in how we have come to understand intellectual disability.

The central concept here is 'aetiology'. In medical discourse this denotes the causes of pathology. Hence, Down syndrome is an aetiological trait seen as leading to intellectual disability: the reason why some people have adaptive behaviour and intelligence deficits is that they have trisomy 21 – an extra chromosome in the 21st pairing which is associated with differing cognitive functions. Aetiology is central in clinical books on intellectual disability. At the same time, these very rarely say anything about *why* this search for explanations is important and worthwhile. In this way, aetiology operates as convention and assumption, something which is presumed to enlighten our understanding of intellectual deficiency but which only occasionally is motivated.

In his introductory book about intellectual disability, Harris (2006:43) provides the assertion that Bourneville 'established' the idea that intellectual disability 'results' from 'brain pathology'. This statement is interesting, as it puts into words many of the assumptions that form the ideology of 'aetiology'. Harris's declaration is premised on two assumptions: *first*, that every pathological state of functioning has an aetiological trait and, *second*, that intellectual disability is, in itself, pathological. Thereby, an important step is taken, from the relative criteria of IQ and adaptive behaviour to deficits in these being deemed 'diseased' and 'sick', which is the meaning of 'pathology'. The idea that intellectual disability results from 'brain pathology' is commonplace in the literature, although not always clearly spelled out. Since aetiology denotes causes of pathology, the pervasive discourse on the importance of clarifying aetiologies implicitly constructs the condition as such as 'pathological'. In addition, as nature is always seen as prior to consciousness and behaviour, the material brain stands as origin and our behaviour as the result of its materiality. Hence, if we presume that all properties of our minds are caused by properties of our brain, then we can postulate that whatever we find strange in human action or behaviour should have a biophysical cause (see Altermark, 2014).

This manner of reasoning plays an important ideological function by displacing the political mechanics operating in the constitution of individuals as 'intellectually disabled'. As was shown above, the diagnosis of intellectual disability is contingent on the judgement that certain ways of functioning are problematic. This judgement must be based on a normative yardstick with regards to the behaviours which are deemed to be requiring a societal response. What aetiology does is to hide such political assumptions and rationales, instead making the correlates found in the brains of individuals masquerade as the real causes of the condition. For example, when we see how dendritic appendages of individuals with Down syndrome are notably different from those of 'normal' people, we believe we have found the 'cause' of their differing cognitive functions. But this requires that we neglect that the rendition of certain differing cognitive functions as 'pathological' underpins the whole exercise; pathology is already a matter of fact when the biological examinations enter to explain the causes of intellectual disability. Thus, when searching for explanations of certain ways of functioning in the brains of certain individuals, we will not find molecular-size labels stating 'pathology'. We cannot *see* or *discover* that some ways of functioning are 'diseased' or 'disordered'. The construction of such labels always exceeds the biological 'facts' of the matter; they are always supplemented by a normative judgement of the examiner. This was the argument of Canguilhem's (1991) analysis of the differentiation between the 'normal' and the 'pathological'; that it must always be made on the backs of normative judgements; that it is always entangled with the values and ideals of a certain social order (see Vailly, 2008:2533). And therefore, we may very well believe that we have found a label of molecular size stating 'pathology' which we can attach to the notably shorter dendritic appendages of individuals with Down syndrome, whilst actually this label was there all along as a presumption.

Corresponding with a central argument from the previous section on classification, the endeavour of finding the biological causes of 'intellectual disability' requires a prior norm concerning what appropriate brain functioning is, and, like before, there is a history to this line of reasoning. Consider, for example, how in an 1869 lecture, Shettle starts off by stating that the definition of aberrant cognition requires a definition of 'health':

> I would describe a healthy mind as that state of the brain, which, existing in any individual, enables him, by a free exercise of the will, to grasp some mental thought or idea; to study some subject which requires considerable exercise of the will of the imagination as well as of the reasoning of the understanding for a considerable time, without wearing its powers; and I would further add, a capability of fixing the attention upon any one subject, or turning it to another at will.
>
> (Shettle, 1869:2)

Only by comparison to this ideal is Shettle able to go on to define mental disease. In the next step, he postulates numerous biological correlates of the unhealthy mind. But these, of course, are not causes of 'mental deficiency'. Rather, the cause of this label is found in his own yardstick of the 'healthy' mind, without which the biological examinations of aberrations would not even be able to take off. Thus, these biological features are not causing unhealthy minds; rather, Shettle's definition of the healthy mind is what produces the search for biological markers. Similarly, in 1905, Mercier stated that any recognition of mental deficiency originates in judgements of behaviour, 'for only by conduct can mind be known' (Mercier, 1905:103). Hence, before the recognition of any biological explanations, there is a recognition that someone has behaved strangely. In the next step of the argument, the causal force of this normative judgement is displaced and masked as biological causality: 'feeling and thoughts, mental states and mental processes, are but the shadows of or accompaniments of a nervous change' (103), leading to the conclusion that 'Whenever [. . .] there is disorder of mind, there must be disorder of nervous processes' (103). Although Mercier explicitly states that judgements of behaviour produce 'mental deficiency', biological scrutiny soon takes over the role of explaining what it is and how it is caused.

The reason why Shettle and Mercier are worth looking into here is because of the apt correspondence to similar lines of reasoning present in current understandings of intellectual disability. Just like then, a judgement of inappropriate behaviour lies at the heart of a diagnosis. Like then, the idea that any behaviour corresponds to properties of the brain leads to the conclusion that there is a cause located in the neuronal organisation of the individual. And like then, this neuronal explanation, whether known or presumed, replaces the normative judgement at the heart of this diagnosis in order to make it appear to be a neutral and scientific fact. Following Butler's (1993:xix–xx) analysis of the materialisation of bodies, the discursive ascription of 'aetiology' thus functions as a further extension of the brains it describes; beyond the reach of social factors, measurement errors, and the critical analysis of power, the blurriness and the historical and social nature of classification are transformed into a question of solid biophysical difference. This is how 'aetiology' naturalises and masks the political investments of the body.

Urla and Terry (1995:1) argue that the idea that social deviancy is expressed on the body is one which reoccurs in Western science and popular thought, from Aristotelian studies of moral expressions of bodies and onwards. Throughout history, people defined by lack of reason and deviant behaviour have represented a fundamental otherness, outside the realm of 'normalcy' and opposite to the idea of the 'good citizen'. However, the separation between this group and 'normal' human beings is far more tenacious than it appears at first glance. Ideas concerning which behaviour constitutes aberrations demanding government responses are historically situated and, as such, fluid and in processes of constant renegotiation. In addition, as was discussed earlier, every quantitative measurement which operates by separating groups will create liminal zones of ambiguity where the boundary between 'normal' and 'abnormal' cannot be clear-cut; the placing of the cutoff point for intellectual disability will inevitably be deemed arbitrary by some, implying that the separation of people with this condition is, in fact, neither 'natural' nor evident. Thus, although people labelled 'intellectually disabled' represent the outside of reason, the line which demarcates this outside is fragile and unclear. Efforts to naturalise intellectual disability by making it a biological fact can be seen as a constant process of answering to this by re-inscribing and protecting the boundary towards 'lack of reason'. And so we forget that the biology of pathology is only searched for *after* deviance is detected, in both a temporal and logical sense; first comes the norm and then the thorough investigation that aims to locate difference in the materiality of the brains of deviating individuals. As Butler (1990:10; 1993:4–7) and Urla and Terry (1995), among others, have argued: mapping the biology and the bodily characteristics of excluded groups has historically served as a method of making judgements of 'otherness' appear as natural and beyond critique. In this way, discourses of 'aetiology' perform the overarching task of projecting deviance onto the body.

The undesirable biology

In close relation to the discourse described earlier, the clinical literature is ingrained with the wider promise of curing intellectual disability. Now, intellectual disability can only be perceived as something to 'prevent' or 'cure' provided the judgement of pathology: of disorder and of something that is best avoided. Thus, it comes as no surprise that both biophysical and social factors understood as 'aetiologies' of intellectual disability are continually talked about in terms of 'risk' and 'risk factors' (see Harris, 2006:79, 103, 116; Carr & O'Reilly, 2007a:23, 45; Carr & O'Reilly, 2007b:52–3; McDermott et al., 2007:7, 22). This structure of reasoning may take the form of detailed lists of potential dangers, associated conditions, and a lack of capacities, which are related to the sub-syndromes of intellectual disability (see Bennett, 2006:342–4; Carr & O'Reilly, 2007b:72–4; AAIDD, 2010:154–5). Taken together, these constitute what social model analysis refers to as a 'tragedy narrative' of disability (Oliver, 1996:32), solely focusing on what people with intellectual disabilities lack and miss.

Rather than isolated mishaps, I argue that this language exposes the biopolitical rationalities underpinning knowledge production on intellectual disability. First, as stated already, conditions labelled 'abnormal' and 'deficient' can only exist when juxtaposed against a prior idea of normality. Secondly, the 'risk' of deviating from this 'norm' constitutes an incentive to act, eugenically, neuroscientifically, or through social politics, depending on which historical epoch and setting we are looking at. Thus, although the science of intellectual disability has developed in terms of its efficiency and its ability to actually help people, there are also important continuities as concerns the dividing line between cognitive ability and disability and its promises of cure and prevention.

To once again return to the argument of Canguilhem (1991), my point here is that the language used to designate 'risks' is bound up with an implicit and presumed normative framework hierarchising ways of being. The favoured existence of 'normalcy' and of 'health' – as opposed to 'disability' and 'pathology' – is today largely implicit, most often figuring as the abstraction that makes a language of 'risk' and 'pathology' possible. In the clinical literature, it is only rarely stated that it is better, more valued, more desirable to have a 'normal' cognition. But without this presumption, it would not make sense to search for 'cures', to propagate 'preventative measures', or to describe an increased likelihood of intellectual disability as a 'risk factor'. Although, there may be answers worth consideration as to why intellectual disability, at least in some cases, should be prevented, for example through decreasing the prenatal alcohol use of pregnant women, the problem is that these questions are not even addressed as normative in the first place. In order to have meaningful discussions about such questions, we need to realise that they are imbued with concerns of government and ideals of how human beings should function.

I want to take a slight historical detour here, to summarise what is implied by this and the previous insights. In 1979, Michael Begab gave his presidential address to the International Association for the Scientific Study of Mental Deficiency (at that time, the largest organisation for researchers of intellectual disability), stating:

> the implementation of knowledge goes well beyond the purview of science and service. Only as we make an impact on the political process and provide

an empirical base for rational decision-making can significant inroads to the global and complex problem of mental retardation be expected.

(Begab, 1979 in Parmeter, 2004:28)

There are two significant things to note in this statement. First, there is a separation, meant to be bridged, between the production of scientific knowledge and politics. Hence, science shall inform politics, ideally, but is not conceived of as 'political' in itself. Similar sentiments seeing scientific knowledge as separate from politics are very much present in the current discussion around disability policy and research (see Shakespeare, 2006:41–2; de Vries & Oliver, 2009; Holland, 2013). Second, Begab denotes 'mental retardation' as a 'problem' that science can help solve, which itself is an expression of the political stakes involved in scientific claims to describe the world. Here, the element of devaluation ('problem') and the element of government ('an empirical base for rational decision making') are enmeshed. Up to this point, this chapter can be read as an analysis of these two interrelated logics; on the one hand, a logic seeking to de-politicise intellectual disability by means of scientific classifications systems and allegedly neutral depictions of the body, and, on the other hand, a logic of knowledge production continuously being interrelated with government, leaning on the prior recognition of intellectual disability as pathology.

As I have argued, what is needed here is the recognition of the primacy of politics. In both a temporal and a logical sense, biological causes are only searched for *after* deviance is detected; it is always preceded by the recognition that there is something abnormal to explain. Hence, I argue that biological correlates or 'causes' of intellectual disability do not prove the natural and pre-political existence of the condition. Rather, they expose that certain 'abnormal' behaviours incite careful scrutiny of the genetic, cerebral, and neuronal features of individuals. Lennard Davis (1995:7) proposes that:

the manner in which this society defines disability in fact creates the category. Able-bodied (or temporarily able-bodied) people safely wall off severely disabled so that they cannot be seen as part of a continuum of physical differences, just as white culture isolates blackness as skin color so as not to account for degrees of melanin production.

As Davis argues, society constitutes disability with reference to norms of the able body and brain. It separates it and distinguishes it, and the process of biologisation that I have examined and discussed here is a central aspect to how this 'walling off', as Davis calls it, is achieved. At the same time, an array of differences and complexities to human cognitive functioning is slated over and sorted into the strict categories of 'normal' and 'deviant'.

In Foucault's analysis, like mine, 'deviancy' exists in a mutually constitutive relationship with what is considered 'normal'. This division has come to shape how we perceive also our own bodies. Lingering at the very heart of this is the dominating ideal of a humanist subject, characterised by reason, rationality, and independence. By projecting shortcomings with respect to this ideal onto the biology of deviants, a difference of sorts is established, a mark of otherness which cannot be escaped, which is natural and thus beyond questioning. For Foucault, this has to do with our desire for authoritative truth, provided by the science of the body that connects individual bodies (and brains, in this case) to modes of regulation, containment, and incitements. Hence, the body is designated as 'origin', as the materiality that cannot be argued against, and as conveying manifest expressions of otherness. It is thereby ascribed a privileged status as source of evidence, understood as 'natural', 'real', and 'authentic'.

The separation of intellectual disability, through classification, however, leads to the threat of what Butler (1993:27) calls 'a terrifying return' of divisions between otherness and normalcy collapsing and of the political investiture in the separation between deviancy and normal becoming exposed. In her analysis of the suppression of queer subjects as a guarding mechanism of compulsory heterosexuality, Butler (1990:23–4) starts from the recognition that normalcy is founded on the separation of several excluded others (see Urla & Terry, 1995). To maintain a strict division between 'male' and 'female', desires that challenge this division must continually be kept at bay from what is considered normal, for example, by understanding them as 'diseased' or 'disordered'. Here, I have analysed a similar guarding mechanism, operating by the discursive structure of 'aetiology', which affirms that 'otherness' is a biological fact, separated from 'normal' cognitive functioning. This is to say that 'aetiology' operates to secure the idea of humanist subjectivity by linking together shortcomings with respect to its ideals with biological markers of the bodies of people seen as deviating.

In conclusion, biological and classificatory knowledge production are mutually reinforcing. Classification cannot detect biological properties, although such are assumed. The depictions analysed above purport to provide precisely this. Biological knowledge, in turn, is premised on a prior presumption of undesirable deviancy of precisely the kind that classification detects and which legitimises the search for causes in the body. The technologies used to segment the population by claiming to detect intellectual disability construct this group to be targeted by socio-political programs and interventions. Thereby, I suggest that the biophysical correlates of intellectual disability, generally understood as the origins of difference, are better regarded as effects of biopolitics and the inclination to locate deviancy in nature.

The politics of biology

The overarching argument up to this point has been that *descriptions* of intellectual disability *constitute* what intellectual disability is. In other words, the knowledge systems that I have analysed create what they propose to represent. More than anything, this necessitates a critical approach to clinical and classificatory depictions in order to make explicit the political rationales of ordering society along the lines of 'normal' and 'pathological' cognitive capacities.

However, doing this, it is also necessary to spell out what is at stake in an analysis of intellectual disability as biopolitics – namely, the very conception of this condition. For the last three decades, the question of whether disability is an individual feature or a social phenomenon or a combination of the two has been a key area of dispute amongst disability theorists. Thus, this chapter is concluded by a discussion of how my analysis relates to this theoretical debate. I will start by discussing the prevailing social and relational models of disability before arguing the case for a conception that transcends the division between nature and politics. Last, I will address and counter some recent critiques of post-structural understandings of disability.

Models of naturalisation

When looked at as a historical instance of resistance, there is no denying that the formation of the social model of disability was important to the disability movement and that it contributed to the abandonment of institutionalisation. In this sense, the activists and scholars that developed this way of approaching disability are an incredible source of inspiration concerning how thinking beyond and acting to change the dominating responses to disability are made possible by means of theory. Still, as the social model itself has become institutionalised in disability studies and has influenced the policy making of the last decades, it also needs to be a legitimate target of critique.

I will argue that the underlying template of the social model, as well as of relational models of disability, are problematic due to their shared assumption that the *biology* of impairment and the *politics* of disability are ontologically separated. As is thoroughly dealt with elsewhere (see Shakespeare, 2006 for an overview), the social model of disability re-conceptualised disability to be interpreted as a social phenomenon, produced by discriminating social structures (see Oliver, 1996). Thus, in contrast to the standard medical thinking on disability, which places the causes of disability in the bodily constitution of the individual, social model analysis sees disability as a result of power relations and social structures. At the heart of this theoretical perspective is the separation between body and social structures, captured by the distinction between bodily *impairment* and socially produced *disability*. By this distinction, this mode of analysis essentially introduced 'disability' as a field of politics, and in this sense, despite the critique that follows, this book is foregrounded by the efforts of this generation of activists and scholars.

As Shakespeare (2006) has pointed out, parallel to the development of the social model(s), a number of related ways of politicising disability gained prominence, which were theorising it as a *relationship* between biological impairment and environmental factors, where the interaction of social factors and impairment produce disability. This way of understanding disability – often labelled 'relational' or 'environmental' – is important since it came to influence many official definitions at the end of the 20th century (see Parmeter, 2004:6; Barnes, 2012:20). For example, a relational understanding is referred to in the 1990 Americans with

Disabilities Act of the US and in the legislations of the Scandinavian countries, it figures in the WHO (2011:4) *World Report on Disability*, where it is dubbed a 'bio-psycho-social model of disability', and it is advanced by UNESCO (Carlson, 2010:6). In classificatory practices this way of conceiving disability has also gained ground, evident for example by how the WHO complements its ICD-10 system with the ICF, which includes social and environmental factors, and in how various editions of the AAIDD (and previously AAMR) conceptualise intellectual disability as an expression of the relationship between individual impairment and environment (Harris, 2006:5, 62; McDermott, 2007:6; Carlson, 2010:6). It is reasonable to understand these relational models as a compromise between hard-line social model analysis and medical conceptions of impairment.

Now, the dominating conceptions of disability – 'social', 'relational', and 'medical' – start from the assumption that the biology of impairment and the social setting surrounding impaired bodies can be analytically separated, which means that the body is never seen as a field of politics. In medical conceptions, as I believe that I have showed throughout this chapter, the body is the cause and focus of interventions; in relational models, the interactions between the distinct entities of 'body' and 'society' results in disability; and in the social model, bodily impairment is seen as prior to but irrelevant for socially produced disabilities. However, considering the arguments that I have offered, disability presents itself as something else; rather than the outcome of social structures solely or of the interaction of body and society, it appears that intellectual disability emerges from a place where the very distinction between nature and politics is suspended. The recognition of certain brains, in their materiality, as 'intellectually disabled', is preceded by the judgement that the materiality of precisely these brains needs to be scrutinised. The search for a cause, for an aetiology, always requires the recognition that something *has been caused*. Otherwise, the dendritic appendages of people with Down syndrome, for example, would only be another bunch of materials inseparable from other properties of the world. What makes this constellation of neuronal organisation matter, and the reason why we set out to scan the brains of people with Down syndrome in the first place, is the social, political, and normative idea that this condition matters and that it is important to find out its causes.

In order to fully develop this train of thought, it is first necessary to specify the critique of the prevailing models of disability. Starting with the social model, although questioning the medical authority over how people with disabilities should live, this conception is unable to question the medical authority to define what impairments *are* – precisely because the bodily constitution is conceived of as prior to politics. Hence, as the social model shifts focus, from individual biology towards discriminatory social structures surrounding the impaired body, the norms that designate certain bodily constitutions as 'disabled' or 'impaired' are rendered outside the scope of criticism. The body is just as naturalised in the social model as it is within medical perspectives – it is just that the proponents of this analysis find it irrelevant to understand 'impairment'. This runs parallel to Butler's intervention into feminist debates regarding the relationship between 'sex' and 'gender'. Butler's (1990:9–12; 1993:xii) argument in this context was that understanding 'gender' as layered on top of biological sex leads to a naturalisation of the sexed biology: what comes to matter in such analyses is the social construction that is inscribed upon biology, but this neglects the becoming of the body through social processes of normatively invested materialisations. In the same way, I argue that the original social model naturalises the impaired body by claiming its political irrelevance. In contrast, I suggest that the impaired/disabled brain, in its materiality, is not thinkable outside a regulative normativity which constitutes our perceptions of certain brains as, precisely, 'impaired' (see Butler, 1993:xii). Furthermore, and contrary to recent formulations of some prominent social model writers (see Barnes, 2012; Oliver, 2007), these are not mere theoretical matters, removed from the lived realities of disability. Rather, approaching the definition of intellectual disability as an instance of biopolitics helps us see that the specification of impairment is an integrated part of how disability politics is organised.

The problem of naturalising the body pertains to the relational model of disability as well: understanding disability as the result of an interaction between impairment and society still leaves out the norms, discourses, and institutions that shape what we understand as 'impairment'. In this conception of disability, the body is primary and analytically separated from 'the social'; it appears before social context and is therefore never seen as a field of politics. Here, society is interacting but never affecting, inscribing, or constructing the impaired biology. This reliance on pre-political impairment makes possible the same structures of naturalisation and de-politicisation of the body that we see in the clinical literature on intellectual disability. It is sometimes suggested that the relational model of disability de-emphasises disability as pathology (Schalock, 2004:382), but what really happens is that it shifts the normative judgement, inherent to labelling something 'pathological', to pertaining to the pre-political body. The 'truth' of disability is thereby thrown into a potentially endless oscillation between nature and culture, biology and social remedies, where both have to be accounted for and understood but where one is always prior and the other always reactive to this primacy. In the end, the attempts to politicise disability by invoking an understanding of its relationship to social organisation bring about a simultaneous *de*-politicisation since they are premised on the naturalisation of the body.

Following Carlson (2010:7), despite the inroads of social perspectives, intellectual disability is still firmly rooted in a biomedical and genetic discourse. One contributing reason for this, I contend, is that the models of disability that have dominated the critique of medicine and psychiatry still end up re-inscribing their ontological placement of human biology in the sphere of nature. Essentially, the on-going debates that revolve around the 'models' of disability are framed by the 'nature–culture' divide, where 'nature' stands for the biology of impairment and 'culture' for the conditions that can enable or disable the biological constitution of the individual. The presumption that the brains of people with intellectual disabilities exist prior to social organisation restricts politics to questions regarding how to accommodate for the natural characteristics of these brains by effective and appropriate social services, as in relational and medical understandings, or to questions about identifying the discriminatory structures that disable individuals, as in social model analysis. The social and relational models of disability may have been necessary to significantly change the pervasive oppression of the 20th century, but their underlying template is insufficient to address the construction of intellectual disability as biopolitics. Thus, rather than a relational or social understanding, my proposal is that we need a critique that starts from the proposition that the body is always already socially constituted.

Beyond 'politics or nature'

In contrast to the debate revolving around the models of disability, I have argued that the constitution of disability is contingent on the ideal of a normal and fully functioning body. This lies at the heart of a biopolitical understanding, for example illustrated by how I showed that this diagnosis has been substantiated with reference to 'normal' cognitive functions. This is also a central theoretical building block of recent attempts of 'cripping' the body. We shall therefore explore the relationship between Crip theory and biopolitics in order to make sense of what a 'cripped' brain might teach us.

First, from a 'Crip' perspective, the implicit or explicit yardstick of normalcy *produces* intellectual disability along the lines of 'able'/'disabled' and operates through a norm system that McRuer (2006:2) has dubbed an ideology of 'able-bodiedness'. Able-bodiedness operates as a non-identity, as the natural order of things, and hence as a presumption that does not need to be explicitly acknowledged (McRuer, 2006:1); it is the invisible and pervasive ideal of how human bodies are supposed to function, instrumental for the formation of all categories defined by bodily and cognitive features. The invisibility of able-bodiedness is why 'normal' cognitive functioning only occasionally is made explicit to define intellectual disability; for the most part, 'normalcy' figures as a shared and taken-for-granted presumption. But it is against this backdrop that it becomes meaningful to discuss certain behaviours as 'abnormal' and to call them 'disorders'. Whilst able-bodiedness/able-brainness is institutionalised as the invisible and normal order of things, disability is operating as its outside, detected, examined, categorised, and named.[2] This also goes for the disabled brain.

Furthermore, since the division between 'normal' and 'disabled' permeates Western societies, there can be no place for anyone outside the distinction between deficient and appropriate cognitive functioning. We are all situated in relation to this division, and it is central to how we appear as subjects (although our relationship to it will only be made explicit once we fail to function as expected; see Goodley, 2014:26). Running alongside Butler's (1990) analysis on heterosexuality as compulsory, McRuer (2006:7) concept 'compulsory able-bodiedness' denotes how we are all impelled to fulfil the ideals of the able body and, I would add, the able brain. Even more closely related to the topic at hand, Clifford Simplican (2015:4) contends that the ideals of political belonging, of being a citizen and democratic subject, function in a similar way as an invisible and unattainable ideal that we are all measured against. In this way – provided that 'intellectual disability' ultimately consists of the perceived failure to be a subject of reason and independence (which we shall get back to in the next chapter) – this diagnosis can be seen as the result of a social ordering along the lines on inside/outside the ideals of humanist subjectivity. In other words: the ideals of able-bodiedness and full functionality compose an ontology of being human, an already existing pre-script as to how we see ourselves and to the ways societies are structured (see Goodley & Runswick-Cole, 2014:4). My critique of knowledge production on intellectual disability has targeted notions that discard this pre-script, that fail to recognise that the knowledge of 'pure' bodies or brains is impossible since it is produced within cultures and discourses that privilege the able brain.

It is important to note that, following Butler's (1990:xxx–xxxii, 26–7) analysis of compulsory heterosexuality, able-bodiedness, as an ideal, operates by being unattainable. Since our functioning will fluctuate throughout life in ways that defy the strict division between 'able' and 'disabled', the perfectly able body, or the perfectly functioning cognition, does not exist; the at-all-times-rational, reasoning, autonomous, and adaptable individual is a fiction that we are nevertheless compelled to accomplish and sustain throughout life. Essentially, this means that there is no identity position of ability in which disability is securely walled off and out of question; we must constantly strive to achieve able-bodiedness, and we must constantly re-inscribe our place in relation to the ability/disability divide through our behaviour (see Goodley, 2014:26). Therefore, the ideal of the able brain is bound to be endlessly repeated on both individual and societal levels. Such repetition is performed through every stage of early detection of deficient cognition: in the milestones checklists that parents judge their kids by, when the preschool or school's psychologists are called in because something 'seems to be wrong', in the 'information talks' provided for parents 'unlucky' enough to have a kid with Down syndrome, and so on. It is also repeated on an individual level as our behaviour is geared towards confirming our proper mental abilities Thus, when Butler (1993:ix) asserts that the materiality of the body – sexed bodies in her analyses, cognitively disabled brains in mine – is constructed through the ritualised repetition of norms, this is what she has in mind; biological constitutions come to matter as 'disabled' through reiterations of certain ways of being as desirable and others as unfavourable that are repeated throughout society and in the behaviour of individuals. In this way, the social and historical processes that have singled out certain characteristics as ordering our understanding of humanity – through the creation of categorisations, taxonomies, but also of lay knowledge and folklore – provide the scene of recognition of some people as 'intellectually disabled' and others as 'normal'. The intellectually disabled brain could not exist without such social and discursive formations.

All of this can be parsed in a more densely theoretical way: irrationality, lunacy, idiocy, foolishness, and so on all figure as the constitutive outside of the 'reason' and 'rationality' of the humanist subject; it is *that* which must be dispelled for the humanist subject to appear as possible. By the same discursive gesture, however, the constitutive outside of reason also appears *within* the dominating normativity, precisely by being its condition of possibility (see Butler, 1993:xiii–xx), which is to suggest that the otherness of cognitive malfunction is latently inside in the form of an unfulfilled possibility figured as threat. The 'threat of a terrifying return' (Butler, 1993:26–7), read this way, is the result of intellectual disability simultaneously being the opposition of and the necessary precondition for the appearance of 'normal' cognitive functioning. The efforts to name, classify, and inscribe the judgement of deviance upon the materiality of the brain are all efforts to enclose otherness, to render it less of a threat, to safely contain it and project it onto the bodies of specific individuals who can be distanced from the humanist subject.

Now, how does this application of performativity relate to the analysis of bio-politics that I have advanced? On the most basic level, of course, biopolitics, as elaborated on by Foucault, is the governing of the population, whilst the primary inspiration I have drawn from Butler (and her theoretical heirs) has been related to understanding the relationship between bodies and politics. For Foucault, bio-politics is fuelled by the need to manage the population. His is an analysis of the concerns of government and the productiveness of power. For Butler and some Crip writers, performativity stems from the need to consolidate identity. This is why the domain of 'abject' beings returns to haunt normalcy: theirs are analyses of how the productiveness of power has come to shape the becoming of embodied subjects, through processes of what Butler calls 'materialisation'. Thus, 'biopoli-tics' has helped us recognise that classification and clinical knowledge are preceded by the recognition that there is a group of people in society that needs to be separated and targeted by government. The analysis of the relationship between biology and politics that draws on Butler, on the other hand, proposes that the differences of people with intellectual disabilities are dependent on the prior recognitions of deviancies – from the same humanist ideals that incite governmental action. In other words, the societal reproduction of ideas which makes certain differences matter are the same processes that governments act on. And in this way, biopolitics helps us explain the rationalities of government, whilst Butler's performativity helps us understand the social constitution and consolidation of biological differences.

In summary, thus, the invention of intellectual disability meant a redisposition in the discursive structure underpinning the humanist subject. During the first decades of the 20th century, this diagnosis came to figure as the opposite of ideals of 'reason' and 'independence', which also meant handling the threat and spectral nature of a constitutive outside. By being inserted into a binary of norm/deviancy, unreason was meant to be enclosed and governed as a way of rendering it less of a threat. Thus, from being an unnameable and unspecified outside, figuring only as a defining absence of the humanist subject, 'intellectual disability' came into being as 'otherness', named and specified in order to be properly excluded and separated from human reason. Now, as totalising – and perhaps pessimistic – as this analysis may seem, a line of reasoning often emphasised in theoretical attempts of 'cripping' disability concerns its potential to trouble our conceptions of 'normalcy' (see McRuer, 2006:10; Goodley & Runswick-Cole, 2014:4). That is, the very instability of the system of signi-fication, formed around 'otherness' and 'norm', implies that there is always room for contestation, resistance, and rethinking. This is what Butler (1993:25) calls the task of refiguring the necessary outside as a future horizon, in which the violence of exclusion is constantly in the process of being overcome. Viewed in this way, the instability of the category of 'disability' can be seen as a resource for critique (see Garland Thomson, 2012), as Goodley and Runswick-Cole (2014:14) points out: to the extent that 'able-bodiedness' operates as a taken-for-granted discursive system of power, disability may very well serve not just as the otherness of this ideal but also as a site of contestation (Goodley & Runswick-Cole, 2014). Like Butler (1990) analysed 'gender trouble', thus, we may follow McRuer (2006:10) asking about the extent to which we are living in a society equally haunted by 'ability trouble'. Indeed, that the construction of intellectual disability requires a continuous process of reiterating a prior devaluation suggests that the biopolitical regime which produces knowledge of this condition is haunted by its own inability to reach systemic closure; the will to normalise, as Garland Thomson (2006:262) calls it, can never be satisfied. We shall return to this discussion, regarding discursive openings and disruptions as possibilities of resistance, in the last three chapters of this book.

Realism strikes back

After the 'linguistic turn' of deconstruction and discourse theory in the social sciences and humanities, 'realism' was bound to regain ground at some point. In the last decade, the materiality of the body (and other physical things) has once again become a locus of social theory. This surge has been noticeable also within disability studies, where prominent scholars such as Tom Shakespeare (2006), Tobin Siebers (2008), and Simo Vehmas (Vehmas & Mäkelä, 2008; Vehmas & Watson, 2014) have called for a return to a biological understandings of impairment, criticising what is perceived as a one-sided focus on discourse and social construction. As a finale to this chapter, I want to finish by addressing these critiques in order to clarify what my position entails.

First, some critics have proposed that Butler's theorisation of subjectivity and the body risks leading to a neglect of the material realities of disability and have warned against a facile translation of 'sex' into 'disability' (Samuels, 2002; Siebers, 2008: 6–7). Along these lines, it has also been suggested that queer/crip analysis reduces disability to a discursive construct that is not 'real', for example indicating that various hardships associated with atypical cognitive functioning can be comprehended as 'mere' social constructions (see Vehmas & Watson, 2014:9). This line of critique, I believe, is unfortunate and represents a grave misrepresentation of Butler's theoretical position; indeed, it is an accusation premised on precisely the division between 'reality' and 'construction' that Butler posits as one of her main targets. Her point is the inseparability of body and society, arguing that what can be understood about the subject and their body is 'set out within the cultural frames of intelligibility' (Taylor, 2013). As has been alluded to, following Butler, the question is not whether intellectual disability exists or not; it is what it means for something to exist and whether the existence of (intellectual) disability is possible to bracket off from the social sphere.

What is implied by Butler's position? As I will argue, certainly not that there are no biological – or other – differences between people that are labelled with intellectual disability and other people. Nevertheless, precisely this has been a regular target of realist critiques, which I will exemplify here with Foley's (2016) to-the-point appraisal of post-structural disability theory. He argues that

> To claim that something is socially constructed is to imply it can be changed. To claim that an intellectual impairment such as Down syndrome is socially constructed is to imply that the cognitive differences this impairment refers to – and which differentiate people with Down syndrome from people without intellectual disability – can be changed and that such differences can be collapsed. That is to say, if we change how society is structured then people with Down syndrome will possess the same cognitive skills as those enjoyed by their contemporaries without intellectual disability. However, as I have proven, such claims are not only false but that the authors who claim to be theorising impairment *qua* impairment are doing no such thing – they are rather theorising the social response to such impairments.
>
> (Foley, 2016:7)

As should be evident from the arguments that I have proposed, although the social responses to people labelled with intellectual disability quite obviously do affect the cognitive capacities of the group to some extent, the point of post-structural disability theory should never be to argue against difference but about coming to terms with that *every* biological constitution could be understood otherwise, indeed, that the designation of biology as being prior to politics itself is a discursive figuration. Hence, the fact that something 'could be changed' does not imply that it can be 'collapsed', as Foley implies, but that its meaning, implications, and treatment could have ended up in other ways. It is not inconceivable to imagine a society in which we would have found no reason to examine the chromosomes of people with Down syndrome, indeed, a society in which this difference, or other differences of cognitive functioning, would not be the basis of classification and categorisation at all. This would of course not erase the extra chromosome in the 21st pairing, but it would arguably mean that Down syndrome would be fundamentally altered as compared with what it is today. Thus, although it is possible that some disability theorists should be more careful in this respect, my argument is not that the differences between, let us say, people diagnosed with Down syndrome and 'normal' people are chimera appearing as 'real' due to 'social constructions' but that the endeavour of naming, scrutinising, interpreting, and thereby *constituting* Down syndrome is inherently social. Again, humanity is composed of an incalculable array of differences – but not all differences matter. Only some differences are interpreted as constitutive, fundamental to what we are, and hence incite medical and psychological scrutiny to map behavioural characteristics and biophysical correlates. The processes that decide exactly which bodies matter in what ways is always culturally embedded and socially invested (Butler, 1993). In parallel to Foley's argument, Vehmas and Mäkelä have argued that the extra chromosome of people with Down syndrome is a 'brute fact', untouched by whatever cultural and social comprehensions of this condition there are. But, as Goodley (2017:135–6) argues in response, pulling this syndrome out of its social, cultural, and political context means ignoring the fact that normative and social judgements – reasonable or not – is the very reason why we started to search the genomics of members of this group in the first place. Hence, the analytical point is not that biological differences do not exist but that they must be *put into existence* to become part of how we perceive the world.

As is evident in the second part of Foley's quote, my line of reasoning, from a realist viewpoint, represents a way of *responding* to the biological fact of impairment rather than exposing its political origins. As he seems to argue, the fact that knowledge about impairments may be socially constructed does not mean that the biological differences are; it is for example logically consistent to both assert that the knowledge systems surrounding intellectual disability are part of an apparatus of power, that everything we know about some syndrome is socially constructed, *and* that the biological differences represented by, say, Down syndrome are pre-political properties of the world. Hence, his argument goes, the fact that knowledge about intellectual disability is social does not mean that its biophysical causes are. Rather paradoxically, thus, Foley and realists of his ilk are accusing post-structuralism of theoretical obscurity through abstraction whilst at the same time hinging their argument on the existence of a body and brain that both can be abstracted from any conceivable social context and from human consciousness as such. In a similar way, Vehmas and Mäkelä (as quoted in Goodley, 2017:134–5) has proposed that 'impairment' can be understood as analogous to mountains, in the sense that 'mountains exist whether we experience them or not'. Peculiarly, thus, biological matter, figured as untouched by human consciousness, has become central to a set of arguments against a social theory of disability. One is indeed hard pressed to find any possible bearing on disability politics of the kind of body that these scholars are bringing about as their argumentative death stroke against post structural theory, since the body prior to discourse, whether we believe in it or not, is politically irrelevant. What matters to politics is how biological features come into being as objects of knowledge for purposes of government; the brains and bodies that do matter in discussions revolving around the politics of intellectual disability are not thought experiments but the stuff that we experience, interpret, form stigmas around, and make the basis of political interventions. Recognising this is to take an epistemological standpoint rather than discussing ontological difference; all instances of biological matter that are touched upon by human consciousness are thus rendered social. Everything that can be said and known about it will be impossible to separate from the sphere of politics. 'The body in itself' that exists independently of it being experienced, perhaps represents a meaningful quandary of metaphysics but should hardly be an issue of disability theory.

More important is the complementing assertion, put forth by Foley (2016) and Vehmas and Watson (2014), that the recognition of disability as socially consti- tuted implies the normative proposition that differences need to be collapsed into sameness. That is, these authors argue that propositions that intellectual disability is a category made up implies that it *ought* to be changed. It is certainly true that such normative propositions are often hidden in allegedly descriptive analyses of how disability is constituted – and I have to admit that I have sometimes fallen prey to it myself (see Altermark, 2014, 2015). However, it does not follow from my analysis that intellectual disability should be abandoned as a diagnosis or that the normative goal is to collapse all categorisations of intellectually disabled people. In their interpretation of 'deconstruction' as an analytical effort to efface all difference, Vehmas and Watson (2014) misinterprets both how Derrida originally used the term and how it was adopted by Butler. For both, deconstruction is an act of 'crossing over' rather than discarding some certain concept, thereby displacing its meaning rather than arguing in favour of simple abandonment. I will develop my ideas concerning the purpose and ethos of this form of critique in the last three chapters of this book. Suffice for now to say that the normative implications of deconstruction are much more modest than what its opponents suggest. Hence, rather than striving for erasure of difference, what I do contend is that we *ought* to consider what a world would look like when help systems, answering to the fluctuating abilities of human beings, were not premised on diagnoses and classifications of disabilities, that is, a world in which the normative devaluation of disability was crossed over and where the norm of the able body and brain was replaced with something else. In his defence of discourse theory against accusations similar to the ones that I have dealt with here, Goodley (2017:135–8) similarly points to the critical potential of theory; it should be a tool for us to destabilise our taken-for-granted notions – not necessarily to abandon them, I would add, but to entertain the possibility that they could be rethought. Provided the track record of the normativity of the able body and brain, the grievances and stigma it has cast against people failing to fit the bill, I do believe that there are good reasons to reconsider what a world without it would look like.

Lastly, realist critiques are often accompanied with the assertion that some impairments (still understood as pre-political facts about the body) – as for example conditions that cause chronic pain or premature death or that severely hamper the possibilities of having a good life – *are indeed reasonable to devalue*. This has for example been a key argument in Shakespeare's (2006:38–43) call for a recognition of the importance of biological impairment in disability theory. There are several aspects to this. First, the very recognition that it is reasonable to see some states of functioning, for example involving severe pain, as undesirable confirms the importance of normative judgements for our understandings of disability. One could reasonably argue that an understanding of severe chronic pain that excludes a negative normative judgement does not present us with an adequate understanding at all. Likewise, a culture that excludes the recognition of the need for a cure for cancer, which is based on the judgement that cancer is bad, has not fully appreciated what cancer is. Normative judgements are thus central to our knowledge about our bodies and brains – whether they are reasonable or not. My point is not that implicit normative judgements are necessarily misguided but that they need to be recognised. When Vehmas and Watson (2014:640) rhetorically ask whether pregnant people eating folic acid are engaged in biopolitics, my immediate answer is that they are and that it undoubtedly is the case that folic acid pills result from normative judgements about intellectual disability – which by itself says nothing about whether recommending or eating folic acid pills is justifiable. The importance of understanding biopolitics, however, is exposed when we consider the opposite scenario, in which we do not attend to the norms and political stakes of various efforts of preventing some lives from coming into being. Should disability studies, for example, ignore the normative judgements involved in pre-natal diagnosis or the norms that once went into eugenics and institutionalisation? Is that really an attractive vision of how disability theory should go about its business?

In summary, the problem of the new realism of impairment and disability politics is that it remains within the confines of the nature/politics divide. But, as I believe that my analysis in this chapter has showed, the purpose of post-structural attempts of theorising the body should be to move beyond this distinction. Disability theorists working in the tradition of thinkers such as Foucault and Butler are pressed to answer whether they believe in the biology prior to discourse and whether they locate specific effects of certain impairments in the material body or in the sphere of social organisation, whilst the point, all along, was to argue that the pure body is a fiction and that the very division between politics and nature is misguided. The general line of criticism, which Foley and Vehmas and Watson have represented here, presses post-structural theory for answers to questions it has never asked.

In the final three chapters of this book, I will develop a conception of intellectual disability that starts from two fundamental dimensions of human vulnerability as concerns how biology interacts with the world and as concerns how these interactions are discursively framed. As we shall see, this analysis resolves many of the tensions that haunt the debates about the ontological status of disability. However, before that, the next three chapters will analyse the central issue of this book: the politics of post-institutionalisation.

Notes

1 Here, there is a range of numbers in the literature, spanning between one-fourth and one-half of those with intellectual disabilities. This depends on when the account was published (as an increasing number of biological correlates are described in the literature) and as concerns whether the statement is made of intellectual disability/'mental retardation' or 'learning disabilities'.
2 As Goodley (2014:23) remarks, this resembles the ways that colonial knowledge is present as neutral and universal through the mobilisation of the vocabulary of humanism, philanthropy, and human rights.

Part II

Citizenship

3 Philosophy

In the previous chapter, I argued that scientific knowledge systems of intellectual disability construct the condition as biologically anchored otherness for the purpose of making the population governable. The three chapters of this second part of the book turn to analyse what the present government of intellectual disability amounts to, how it operates, which rationalities it is underpinned by, and to what effects for labelled people. In other words, I will examine the citizenship politics of post-institutionalisation.

To summarise what will be presented in this and the coming chapters: the analysis will revolve around a recurring structure – in fundamental ways, intellectual disability causes *disruptions* to common notions of that which defines human beings and their societal belonging. Disruption means that schemes of justice, morality, or politics are destabilised when faced with a group that is presumed to be different with respect to what is understood as characterising a human being. This is to say that whenever a political project makes reason and autonomy a basic presumption, and as long as intellectual disability is seen as lacking in this respect, the resulting disruptions must be resolved by some sort of *supplement* in order to deal with this condition. Supplements can consist, for example, of charity or segregation, but also of special attempts to include the group without reconsidering the humanist subject; a supplement is an extra principle necessary to deal with what falls outside of the ordinary.

In this and the following two chapters, I will argue that attempts to include people with intellectual disabilities are destined to repeat exclusion as long as they are founded on the same ontology of human beings which produced the otherness of the condition in the first place; such attempts will be entrenched by the structure of disruption and supplementation. The arguments of the previous chapter are necessary to understand this; the notions of human reason put forward by Locke and Kant heavily influenced early conceptions of intelligence, IQ testing, and the emerging field of psychology, all dedicated to identifying this group as falling outside the scope of 'normal' humanity. Today, notions of citizenship that are ingrained by the very same tradition of humanist philosophy, defining the group by what they lack, are meant to include this group. As I will show, the effect of this is that contemporary politics of intellectual disability govern both by including and by re-inscribing exclusion; it is a dual way of managing that both seeks to create a new included citizen-subject whilst upholding otherness through maintaining the marginalisation and restrained agency of people with this condition. The concurrency of these two modes of government defines the post-institutionalisation era; the disruptions of politics of inclusion caused by intellectual disability is supplemented by efforts that maintain their exclusion whilst fashioning them to become normative citizens.

In important ways, this analysis breaks with prevailing ideas about disability politics as developing progressively, from oppressive rule of institutionalisation towards politics of citizenship. Firstly, when the politics of inclusion operates as intended, it moulds subjectivity and creates citizen-subjects (see Cruikshank, 1999). Hence, 'inclusion' is a means of government, an instance of biopolitics that works through 'the conduct of conduct' (Foucault, 2000:341; 2007), rather than lack of state power. As my analysis will show, particularly in Chapter 5, the absence of force and coercion does not mean the absence of government and policy commitments to 'citizenship', and 'inclusion' does not imply the withdrawal of the state. Secondly, government by inclusion is parallel to and intertwined with systematised and structural exclusions of a kind that are commonly associated with institutionalisation. Thus, intellectual disability remains the constitutive outside of citizenship ideals, also after the advent of politics of inclusion.

I will develop these arguments with respect to three different analytical levels and empirical sources. First, this chapter is a political theoretical critique in which I engage with the arguments of a number of prominent philosophers. The next chapter is a discourse analysis of a number of treaties and international policy documents in which I analyse their presumptions and discursive implications. Lastly, Chapter 5 is based on an interview study in which I analyse how support workers describe their job in order to understand the group home as a place where citizens with intellectual disability are both produced and constrained. I will show how the structures of disruption and supplement and of inclusion/exclusion run through all of these arenas of intellectual disability politics.

To get these arguments going, it must first be remembered that ideas of citizenship have a history; this notion of societal belonging is founded on conceptions of 'independence', 'autonomy', and 'participation' which have been central to Western political thought. In this chapter, I will trace the history of these concepts with respect to intellectual disability, showing that the historical exclusion of this group is a result of how its members have always been seen as lacking the fundamental capacities that our notions of full belonging and self-ownership are founded on. In other words, to understand the politics of post-institutionalisation, it is necessary to look at why people with intellectual disabilities became outsiders in the first place. I will start by discussing the otherness of intellectual disability in John Locke's *Two Treatises of Government* (1988 [1690]), David Hume's *An Enquiry Concerning the Principles of Morals* (1957 [1751] i.e. '2:d Enquiry'), John Stuart Mill's and Harriet Taylor's *On Liberty* (2003 [1899]), and the moral philosophy of Immanuel Kant, primarily as developed in *Groundwork of the Metaphysic of Morals* (2002 [1785]). The selection of these works is purposely diverse: my argument is that 'deficient intelligence' has operated as a grounds for exclusion in similar ways across Western political thinking. This is the heritage Enlightenment philosophy leaves us with; it is the legacy of the humanist subject. As my argument will be that the relegation of people with intellectual disabilities is more than mere historical prejudice, I will then discuss John Rawls's (1971) theory of 'justice as fairness', which explicitly discards people with cognitive deficits from the conception of justice. In summary, the first half of this chapter shows why intellectual disability and citizenship make an odd couple; the history of citizenship has been premised on the exclusion of people seen as lacking reason and rationality.

In turn, in the second half of the chapter, I will go on to argue that attempts to remedy the exclusion of intellectual disability will fail to the extent they re-inscribe the humanist subject. In parallel to what we will encounter in the coming two chapters, efforts to include members of this group that proceed from conceptions of societal belonging founded on reason and autonomy are also destined to maintain exclusion. Here, I will discuss Charles Taylor's notion of a politics of recognition and thereafter Martha Nussbaum's capabilities approach. Nussbaum and Taylor are both chosen because they explicitly address inclusion of people with intellectual disabilities.[1] This discussion will then be of great help when we turn to analyse the complexities of policy attempts to target people with intellectual disabilities with politics of inclusion.

Excluding lack of reason

To start with: if we take 'citizenship' to denote the relationship between the individual and the political community, it becomes evident that certain classes of people, specified by their inferior minds, recur throughout the history of philosophy as the constitutive outside of societal belonging. Consider the examples that follow.

The *Second Treatise of Government* contains an intriguing critique of Filmer's notion of absolute patriarchal hierarchy and rule, whereas John Locke (1988) uses the potential for reason in children as grounds for contesting the absoluteness of patriarchal rule. Since children have this potential, the authority over them is not absolute but restricted until 'reason' has developed. Locke then goes on to contrast the temporary control of children with the rule of people suffering from a permanent lack of reason (Locke, 1988:308); the 'lunaticks' and 'ideots' who by merit of their deficient minds cannot be part of the social contract. In other words, and as we shall get back to in a moment, lack of reason *disrupts* Locke's theory of the contract, which requires a *supplement* consisting of 'permanent patriarchal rule' of the permanently deficient. This shows how deficient rational capacities mark the limits of inclusion for Locke's social contract.

David Hume, in the 2:d Inquiry (1957), differentiates between a government of justice and a government of a principle of charity, explicitly stating that those of 'inferior strength, both of body and mind' shall be subjected to the principle of 'gentle usage' rather than to a 'government of justice'. Hume bases his conception of justice on what he calls 'rough equality', which means that people must have similar capabilities for situations of societal cooperation – and hence justice – to arise (see Nussbaum, 2006:47, 61–2). He calls the conditions for such cooperation 'circumstances of justice', and the gist of his argument is that men will only work out principles to govern themselves if they believe that others have similar capacities. Although Hume does not base his theory on the idea of a social contract, his 'circumstances of justice' resemble the structure of Locke's motivations for excluding people who fail to meet the ideals of mental capacity.

Finally, in their ardent defence of diversity and tolerance in *On Liberty*, John Stuart Mill and Harriet Taylor (Mill, 2003 [1899])[2] exempt from their principles of liberty people who lack reason. Their discussion of the perpetual tension between the sovereignty of the individual and the oppression of the state concludes with a defence of the absolute independence of each in matters which only concern themselves (Mill, 2003:81). This principle, however, is disrupted a few lines later by people not 'in the maturity of their faculties' for whom such individual freedom does not apply (Mill, 2003:81). Mill and Taylor are talking not only about children and legal minors in this context but also about those who need to be taken care of by others due to their lack of reason (Mill, 2003:81). Thus, dependency and mental inferiority are here intertwined. Accordingly, the principles of freedom and individual sovereignty can only be granted for *all* if simultaneously held back from *some*, illustrating how tolerance and diversity, so central to Mill and Taylor's argument of individual freedom, are demarcated by a presumed set of capacities that not all people possess. Echoing Locke and Hume, the capacity of reason operates both as an underlying ontology of humanity and as a dividing line between what is inside and what is outside of the sphere of inclusion.

It might be suggested that these examples, at least to a degree, are the result of the historical settings of these philosophers. In a trivial sense, this is certainly correct. However, for my purposes it is also beside the point. I am not interested in charging a bunch of historical figures with 'ableism'. Rather, in order to historicise our present, I want to explore how the Western history of political thinking is structured by an ontology of human beings which produces exclusions; I am interested in how humanism, as a way of seeking to define human existence by singling out certain characteristics, has always been bounded. This history is inscribed onto our present: the paradoxical simultaneity of inclusion and exclusion that characterises present intellectual disability politics must be understood against the backdrop of how our conceptions of belonging have been premised on excluding people who are assumed to lack reason.

Reason and exclusion

The exclusion of persons 'lacking reason' from notions of belonging is founded on a specific understanding of society and on a related conception of the subject. To illustrate this, I will turn to two of the most influential philosophers in each area: John Locke and his idea of society as founded on a social contract and the subject of Immanuel Kant's moral philosophy. Although not all Western political theories of modernity are contractual and not all notions of subjectivity are

Kantian, I do believe that these two examples are helpful to pinpoint why Western philosophy has excluded people defined as intellectually deficient.

The previous reference to Locke's justification of patriarchal rule serves as an illustration of his more general treatment of intellectual disability. In what I consider to be the best analysis of intellectual disability and the history of Western political philosophy, Clifford Simplican (2015) argues that Locke's exclusion of 'mental deficiency' is pivotal to his overarching political project. Following her argument, the social contract establishes an ideal, which is also deeply ingrained in present societies, concerning what political participation requires. Thus, when Locke argues that people 'born [. . .] to the use of the same faculties' should be equal in regards to the state, he sets a precedent for how political philosophy, within and outside the contract tradition, has premised political rights and duties on certain capacities (see Clifford Simplican, 2015:26). In turn, this implies that some people, on these grounds, are excluded. Locke frequently uses 'idiots', along with other denotations of 'mental deficiency', to limit the sphere of political membership (Clifford Simplican, 2015:25–7). In his argument, such people serve the purpose of characterising 'normal' personhood by exemplifying abnormality. Through a close reading of Locke's essay, Clifford Simplican (2015:33) convincingly argues that impediments of reason are vital to Locke's political theory, whose notion of humanity is ultimately rooted in the idea that reason is the faculty that comes closest to God's imperfectability. In turn, she therefore argues that an understanding of Locke's social contract requires that we acknowledge how it is premised on an implicit 'capacity contract' that states that membership in society hinges on the rational capacities of individuals (Clifford Simplican, 2015:40–1). By the capacity contract, 'reason' operates as an implicit justification of political subordination, and in this way, Locke can justify political rule on the grounds of the mental faculties of those subjected to government (see Clifford Simplican, 2015:40).

Although Clifford Simplican's argument has much more nuance, arguing that the 'capacity contract' also stresses a form of human vulnerability that can be mobilised for the purposes of solidarity, it is the exclusion of unreason and the supplementary addition of patriarchal rule that are important for my purposes. People need to be removed from political membership in order for Locke's political theory and notion of personhood to take off. Now, if the social contract were to offer a story of society whose main actor is a subject characterised by rational capacities, Immanuel Kant could be seen as the central philosopher who developed this notion of subjectivity by making it the basis of his moral philosophy.[3] Understanding the prerequisites of being included in Kant's conception of 'moral autonomy' can thus help us to understand the primacy of reason in modern philosophy more generally.

For Kant, individual autonomy means consolidation with a universal moral law: we can all be moral in the same way since our individual rationality leads us down the same path of reason. Thus, autonomy and reason are tightly knit together. An important component of this argument is that 'reason' should be conceived of as functioning *a priori*, that is, as prior and separate from any experiences,

senses, and observations (Kant, 2002:4–5); the moral law is established by turning inwards and seeking out principles by means of pure rationality, an exercise
that discards our sensory impressions and social ties from moral deliberation. This
means that, although reason will provide all moral agents the same answers, the
exercise of deriving the moral law is strictly individual.

Kant's (2002:46–7) most famous moral dictum is found in his second formulation of the categorical imperative, stating that we should never treat others as
mere instruments but also always as ends in themselves. This principle has been
central to liberal philosophy, for example seen in Rawls's notion of justice, in
Nussbaum's capabilities approach, and in various charges against utilitarianism.
For Kant, this principle means that we should acknowledge that the rational wills
of others can be in agreement with ours and be able to contain in themselves the
ends of our actions (2002:47–8). Thus, the principle effectively ties the universality of individual reason to a set of moral requirements towards others. Kant
deduces from this that respect for other human beings, in the strongest sense of the
word 'respect', is a respect for their capacity to be moral – it is to acknowledge in
others a morality that is guided by reason. Since we cannot force our moral views
upon others, and since actions that are forced do not qualify as 'moral', the notion
of the universality of reason serves to derive communality in a world inhabited
by autonomous selves. What makes actions moral is that they are anchored in the
exercise of individual deliberation. Hence, Kant's moral philosophy is deontolog-
ical, which means that consequences are irrelevant to moral evaluations of actions
(Kant, 2002:16). It follows that there is a distinction between acting from *one's
own recognition* of moral laws and *in accordance* with moral laws (for example
due to custom or legislation) even though the actual course of action may be the
same. Motivation rather than results is what makes actions right or wrong. For
Kant, the enforcement of judicial laws serves the purpose of ensuring that the
actions of individuals conform to what is morally required even in the absence of
a moral motivation. However, only human rationality can render actions moral,
which means that behaviour conforming to moral principles but produced by
custom or legal measures does not deserve the respect and dignity reserved for
behaviour derived by *a priori* deliberation (see Honig, 1993:26). Therefore, those
who lack the will of the moral law – that is, who lack 'reason' – are excluded from
the moral community and figure in society purely as subjects of laws that serve
to protect the circumstances of moral reasoning for the fully rational part of the
population.

Hence, a precondition for being respected by others as an autonomous moral
agent is that one possesses the capacity to derive the moral law by reason (Kant,
2002:17). Of course, reason is not the only characteristic of human beings, but it
is the characteristic which sets us apart from other living things: although humans
also have needs, desires, and instincts, being moral is about raising ourselves
above these by establishing laws for our own actions (see Nussbaum, 2006:131). In
this way, Kant depicts a subject split between 'animality' and 'rationality', where
being moral consists of taming the former by the latter. Through doing this, Kant
locates those failing to meet his rigorous standards of reason outside the sphere of

moral capacity, and in this way, the formation of a grounds for belonging – here, to a moral community – produces a simultaneous set of exclusions of those that are perceived as deficient (see Honig, 1993:18–19, 38–41).

To summarise, the architecture of exclusion in Kant corresponds to Locke's 'permanent patriarchal rule' and Hume's earlier-mentioned principle of 'gentle usage'. The motivation behind Locke's subjection of individuals seen as cognitively inferior to 'patriarchal rule' is that these fail to meet the requirements of what is distinctively human. Likewise, in Hume, those inferior in 'body and mind' cannot be subjects of justice precisely because they fail to conform to the idea of what it is being fully human. Obviously, the designation of reason and rationality as what characterises humans take different forms in Kant, Locke, and Hume. However, all of them share such ontological commitments to human nature that correspondingly constitutes certain individuals as Others. These examples are all pointing towards the same fundamental fact: there is a yardstick of what defines humanity, ingrained in the philosophical history of citizenship and societal belonging, which is disrupted when confronted with people falling below the bar. As was seen in the previous chapter, the linkage between philosophy and judgements of pathology exposes how the conception of the 'fully human' is what institutes diagnosis of people perceived as lacking intelligence. The history of the philosophy of citizenship and its understanding of reason as the defining characteristic of humans is also a history of government.

Rawls's justice as fairness

It is important to note that the relationship between reason and exclusion is much more than a historical artefact but rather a structure that recurs in political thinking that starts from a definition of personhood as reason, autonomy, or deliberation. In what follows, I will discuss the structure of disruption and supplement in the philosophy of John Rawls, who for similar reasons as Locke, Kant, and Hume explicitly excludes people with intellectual disabilities from his conception of justice.

Rawls's *A Theory of Justice* (1971) is arguably the most influential book of political philosophy of the 20th century, reconceptualising social contract theory and building on Kant's moral philosophy and Hume's 'circumstances of justice'. Rawls's exclusion of people with deficient cognitive capacities follows from his assertion that the 'sense of justice' is a mental capacity involving the exercise of thought (1971:11). Although a contract theory, Rawls's idea differs from classical contractarian thinking in that he does not figure a state of nature from where the contracting parties create political order. Instead, his original position is to be conceived of as a fictive situation that works as a procedural legitimisation of principles of justice. The only assumptions made about the characteristics of the contracting parties in the situation in which the contract is agreed upon – what he calls the 'original position' – are that their intellectual abilities lie within the 'normal range' and that they are acting out of self-interest (Rawls, 1971:10, 83–4). Hence, rather than deriving the principles of justice from characteristics of the individuals that enter into the contract or from pre-societal natural rights, a set of restrictions of the contracting situation itself is what produces his principles of justice. The gist of his argument is that, in a situation in which individuals do not know what kind of person they will become and what kind of life they will live in an unknown future society – that is, behind a 'veil of ignorance' – two principles will be chosen to govern society: (1) that each person has a an equal right to the most extensive liberty that is compatible with a similar liberty for others and (2) that the only tolerable inequalities deviating from equal distribution are of such a nature that the least well off in society gains from them (Rawls, 1971:53, 266–7).

The question here is why Rawls needs to exclude people falling outside the normal range of abilities from the contracting situation. A first reason is his assumption that contracting parties are motivated by mutual advantage. Following Rawls's assumptions, for a solely self-interested person there would be no purpose in making a contract with people who are unlikely to contribute to the common good. Hence, provided this assumption, Rawls deduces that people who are likely to demand extensive care and leave few contributions would be unwelcome behind the veil of ignorance (see Nussbaum, 2006:104, 117). At this stage of his argument, Rawls (1971:109–10) leans heavily on Hume's 'circumstances of justice', mentioned earlier, which hold that concerns of justice emerge between people of roughly equal capacities in a world of scarce resources. As contracting parties are not allowed to be motivated by benevolence,[4] people with disabilities are left out of the contracting situation. A related motif here, pointed out by Nussbaum (2006:114), is that adding functional limitations to the characteristics of contracting parties would complicate measurements of whether individuals are more or less well off in the future society. For example, two people, one with and one without a disability, can be of similar rank and have similar income, but it would still be hard to say that their situations are comparable. From Rawls's viewpoint, this is problematic considering the second principle of justice, called the 'difference principle', which requires that questions concerning who is more or less well off can be clearly answered. Excluding disability thus means keeping issues of who gains and who does not purposefully simple.

More fundamentally, I believe, Rawls's notion of personhood draws heavily on the rationalism of Kant, with its emphasis on the deliberative capacities of individuals. Indeed, the exercise of deriving principles of justice by discarding one's social roles behind a veil of ignorance can be seen as parallel to the Kantian moral requirements of *a priori* moral reasoning: in both cases, principles of justice or morals are reached by the intellectual exercise of stripping oneself of one's social belongings. The subject projected behind the 'veil of ignorance' functions by deliberative rationality, a subject assumed to be able to turn their back against society to find out what to do and who they want to be: it is a coherent, autonomous, and rational self that reaffirms the principles of justice. The rational subject, in turn, is a guarantee that the contracting parties really choose rational principles from the original position, and thereby the exclusion of intellectual disability is central to ensure the linkage between Rawls's original position and the principles of justice.

Thus, intellectual disability disrupts Rawls's notions of personhood and mutual advantage, which, in turn, means that the handling of this group requires a supplement. Like other contract philosophers, Rawls assumes that those who decide on the principles of the contract and those that these principles apply to are the same: as people with intellectual disabilities are left out of the contracting situation, they are not targeted by its outcome (see Nussbaum, 2006:16). Rawls's solution is to postpone the treatment of people with intellectual disabilities until after the contracting parties have agreed upon the principles of justice, that is, their situation should be handled *ad hoc* through legal arrangements outside the scope of justice. This exclusion is repeated throughout Rawls's work – for example, in the postulation that the contracting parties know that their 'native endowments' all lie within 'the normal range' (Rawls, 1971:83–4); in the statement that the principle aim of the theory is 'to specify the fair terms of cooperation among persons' within a 'normal span of native endowments' (Rawls, 1993:183); and in the assumption that 'persons as citizens have all the capacities that enable them to be cooperating members of society' (Rawls, 1993:20). However, as Clifford Simplican (2015:73, 84) argues, accepting Rawls's own description of this as a mere 'postponement' underplays the perpetual definitional work performed by intellectual disability in his theory of justice. Rawls frequently uses people of inferior intellect – described as subjects of pity and unfortunate circumstances – to demarcate political subjectivity in ways resembling how Locke used 'idiocy' to construct a definition of personhood. Only by discarding certain ways of being can the rational subject be designated as the agent that agrees on the principles of the just society.

Thus, Rawls seeks to discard situations of potential conflict from his theory (see Honig, 1993:127), his deliberative rationality produces flourishing pluralistic societies because all rational and self-interested individuals will choose the same principles of justice. Therefore, people that might not be rational in this way pose a major threat to the homogeneity of the just society, which ultimately explains their exclusion from the original position. And in this way, Rawls continues the tradition of excluding people not conforming to the humanist ideals since they disrupt its ontology of personhood.

Including otherness

To understand the politics of post-institutionalisation, knowing that people with intellectual disabilities have been excluded is not nearly as important as knowing *why* they have been. This is so for reasons already discussed; the efforts to include by citizenship seem to repeat the exclusion of intellectual disability. In other words, the humanist notion of reason and rationality as grounding personhood is both the origin of and cure to exclusion. This becomes evident when we look at theoretical efforts to remedy the exclusions of this group in liberal and Enlightenment philosophy, but that starts from the same ontology of the subject. Hence, below, I will argue that both Taylor's and Nussbaum's versions of inclusion also repeat the exclusion of people with intellectual disabilities because they still, in important senses, commit to the humanism and universalism that constituted the otherness of this group in the first place. Both Taylor and Nussbaum are founding their notions of what characterises humanity in qualities that they also assume that (at least some) people with intellectual disabilities lack.

Recognising intellectual disability

The politics of recognition is one of the prime contenders to liberalism and social contract theory, challenging both assumptions of an autonomous and rational subject and substantial political ideals of liberal justice. It may therefore seem as though Taylor's attempt to include intellectual disability has the potential to lead beyond the earlier-discussed problems. The origin of Taylor's argument is found in Hegel's idea of humans as becoming through mutual recognition. This proposition was largely formulated in opposition to the atomism and pre-social individuals of Kant's moral philosophy. It is also from Hegel's notion of recognition that some of the most piercing criticisms of liberalism have been developed. In his essay 'Politics of Recognition' Taylor (1995) advances the argument that minority cultures ought to be acknowledged as valuable by the dominant culture in dialogical processes of recognition. Theorising colonial practices of subjugation, he argues that a recurring tool in the history of oppression consists of the imposition of negative self-images on the colonised (see Taylor, 1995:65–6). The politics of recognition, therefore, starts with transforming how people view themselves by building mutual respect between different groups and individuals. It follows that, for Taylor, the relationship between individuals and the community is essentially dialogical, whereas other individuals and groups of individuals are preconditions of our self-images and self-understanding. Rather than the self-constituting individual of liberalism, Taylor's proposal focuses on how societies can enable processes of mutual recognition in order to shape identity.

Taylor confronts the otherness of intellectual disability when he seeks to provide a basis for what it is that should be recognised in others. He writes,

> this [universal human] potential, rather than anything a person may have made of it, is what ensures that each person deserves respect. Our sense of the importance of this potentiality reaches so far that we extend it even to people who through some circumstance that has befallen them are incapable of realizing their potential in the normal way – handicapped people, or those in coma, for instance.
>
> (1995: 41–2)

As Taylor presents his argument, he suggests that 'handicapped people', itself a pejorative term, are to be recognised not for what they are but for what they 'potentially' could have been (see Arneil, 2009). Unfulfilled potential, in turn, is the result of special circumstances that 'befall' individuals, meaning that they cannot realise their potential in a 'normal way'. Thus, what makes it possible to include 'handicapped' people in the sphere of recognition is a shift: from an *actual* ability to realise one's potential to having a *potential* for this, although something has prevented it from developing. The word 'even' is important here, indicating that the invocation of 'potential' enables the inclusion of an unlikely candidate. Furthermore, the argument hinges on a differentiation between 'normal' and 'abnormal' ways of realising one's potential, where it is clear that the former is preferable. From this we can conclude that people with intellectual disabilities (together with people in comas) represent something that requires a special measure in order to accomplish inclusion by recognition; although the overarching ethos of the politics of recognition is that it grants respect for individuals based on what they truly are, this principle does not apply to people with intellectual disabilities, who should instead be respected for what they *are not* but once had the potential to become.

To understand how Taylor reaches this conclusion, it is necessary to examine his indebtedness to the Kantian notion of respect. Taylor develops his concept of recognition from Hegel, but it is the influences of Kant that explain the problems with this particular argument. As Taylor (1995:41) notes on the page before the section quoted earlier, and as I discussed a few pages back, for Kant (2002:16–17) it is the capacity to derive moral laws by the faculties of reason that commands from us a sense of respect. What is important here is the shift that Taylor (1995:41) makes when going from Kantian respect of 'reason' to his own proposition of respect of 'potential of reason'. By making this shift, Taylor shows that he believes that he is able to extend recognition 'even' to people with disabilities, which would have been impossible if one used Kant as a jumping-off point. In doing this, Taylor produces a new division, this time between those that can be recognised as moral subjects and those that only are recognised as holding the unfulfilled potential of being moral subjects. An unspoken normativity is thereby operating, in which the actual realisation of Kantian reason is the norm and starting point, while potential as grounds for recognition is the supplementary tool which enables the marginal case to be included. This normativity is made explicit as Taylor states that people with disabilities cannot reach their potential 'the normal way'. Hence, in his efforts to produce a grounds for recognition that includes 'even handicapped people', he simultaneously produces a new line of demarcation between rational subjects and people who merely have the potential to be rational. In this way, the exclusion of Kant is handled whilst also being reproduced.

To fully grasp the implications of this, I want to broaden the perspective to discuss Taylor's reasoning on disability in light of his overarching philosophical project. Markell (2003) has interpreted the politics of recognition as grounded in an idea of sovereignty as temporality, ultimately seeking to secure the future of one's identity. Similarly, Fareld (2008:163–8) argues that Taylor's reading of Hegel ultimately seeks to confirm an already-there stable and coherent identity that is to be re-valued rather than challenged or transformed. This limits the constitutive force of 'recognition' that, at first glance, appears to be central to Taylor's viewpoint (and that certainly was for Hegel). In fact, Taylor presents us with a rather conservative reading of Hegel which ends up close to the assumptions of a true inner identity and of a subject exercising self-mastery, which he originally set out to challenge. Following Fareld (2008:156–7), Taylor thus places the identity of self on a collective level that becomes as un-reflected and taken for granted as the liberal atomistic individual he seeks to escape. What differentiates recognition from misrecognition in Taylor's argument is that the former makes possible the return to a true self that enables different identities to live together in harmonious coexistence. In this way, the figuring of a unified identity is very important for Taylor's larger project of advancing a conception of the value of diversity. Taylor understands differences as being constitutive parts of a united whole and, as long as people are respected and recognised for who they really are, such differences can coexist, nourish each other, and allow citizens to live together peacefully. Diversity thereby translates into the richness of humanity, which means that we all have an interest in the difference of others, since such differences complement our own restricted share of what it means to be human (see Taylor, 1995:72–3). Thus, we all need to be recognised not to become subjects in the first place but to live in peace together (Fareld, 2008:160).

Brought to bear on intellectual disability, by Taylor's argument, this group can be seen as a difference that enriches the whole of humanity, which, in turn, serves as a source of their recognition. However, as it is their *potential* for being rational that should be respected, this simultaneously means that the differences of this group are neglected. The logic of Taylor's argument is that disparities of identity are underpinned by a notion of sameness consisting of the common humanity that diversity provides value to. It is precisely here, I argue, that we have come full circle and are faced, once again, with Kantian respect for persons as respect for their rational capacities. In the end, this is what Taylor (1995:41) uses to knit diversity together into a united whole, the 'universally human' that his theory of recognition cannot do without and which serves as a grounds for the enriching differences of humanity to be layered upon. By ascribing a *potential* of being respected for one's reason to the intellectually disabled, however, Taylor's insistence on an underlying sameness comes at the price of re-inscribing difference, conceived of in a way that looks very much like his own conception of misrecognition. And in this way, Taylor's lingering commitment to a notion of rationality as defining humanity – fulfilled or as potential – both includes and excludes intellectual disability.

The capabilities approach

Whilst Taylor explicitly contests liberal conceptions of membership in political community, Martha Nussbaum (2006:3) proposes her capabilities approach as part of political liberalism and as close to, although criticising, Rawls's theory of justice. She first developed her version of the capabilities approach in *Women and Human Development* (2000), where she argues that basic requirements of justice consist of guaranteeing a minimum level of 10 capabilities which are central to a dignified human life, and the book analysed here – *Frontiers of Justice* (2006) – develops from this earlier work. Among philosophers of disability, Nussbaum provides one of the leading efforts to formulate a grounds for inclusion of intellectual disability. I will therefore present a rather extended and detailed treatment of her argument.

Among Nussbaum's capabilities we find being able to live 'a human life of normal length', being able to have 'good health', being able to 'live towards and with others', and 'being able to form a conception of the good' (Nussbaum, 2006:76–8). As is clear from her formulation of capabilities, it is what people are actually able to do which is important in matters of justice (Nussbaum, 2006:70). The capabilities are understood as un-exchangeable and intrinsically desirable, which means that an increased level of one capability cannot compensate for the lack of any other (175). Government therefore needs to make sure that every citizen reaches a minimum level of each capability, or they have failed to meet basic requirements of justice. As soon as all threshold levels are met, the capabilities approach does not address further issues of distribution, and, in this sense, Nussbaum only offers a limited account of justice. While *Women and Human Development* argues against utilitarianism, slanted in the tradition of economics, *Frontiers of Justice* discusses, adds to, and intensely criticises Rawls's theory of justice. The book reproaches three significant problems of Rawls's theory: its inability to address justice for people with disabilities, global justice, and the justice of non-human animals, stating that the capabilities approach is better suited to deal with all of these. Of course, the treatment of justice for people with disabilities will be the focus here.

First, I want to point out that I believe that Nussbaum is correct: her approach certainly appears to be a better account of justice for people with disabilities than 'justice as fairness'. In addition, as a grounds for formulating political demands concerning disability politics, Nussbaum provides many appealing suggestions that avoid some of the dangers of the social contract tradition. Thus, the following discussion should not be read as a rejection of the capabilities approach as a practical tool to raise political demands. Rather, my treatment of Nussbaum relates to the overarching argument of this chapter, proposing that the inclusion achieved by the capabilities approach, despite its strengths, simultaneously re-inscribes exclusion.

Nussbaum's criticism of Rawls is similar to mine (although she parses her argument in the crisp and seductively clear language of analytical Anglo-Saxon philosophy): the theory of justice excludes 'mental impairment' because it starts from a narrow conception of mutual advantage and because it takes for granted a Kantian notion of personhood as grounded in rationality. I have no major objections here. However, her positioning of the capabilities approach in relation to Rawls is notoriously ambiguous in what I believe to be an analytically significant way. At the opening of the book, she states that justice as fairness suffers from structural problems and that we must rethink what a citizen is and could be in light of her capabilities approach (2006:1–2). She later argues that Rawls is constrained by his adherence to theories of the social contract (57), that the flaw of not being able to handle (intellectual) disability goes directly into the architecture of Rawlsian justice (1, 98), and that these are not merely problems of incompleteness but that they misdirect his basic concerns of justice (4, 139–40). These (and other) formulations suggest a thorough criticism of Rawls and contract theory. On the other hand, Nussbaum continuously points out that she does not intend to dismiss Rawls or the social contract and that she sees justice as fairness and her own approach as allied theories of political liberalism (Nussbaum, 2006:24, 94–5). In her most thoroughly developed formulations, Nussbaum states that the capabilities approach is an extension of Rawls but starts from similar intuitions (120) and that her conception of capabilities takes us further within the three specific areas that her book focuses on (69, 94–5), implying that she believes that justice as fairness provides satisfying answers in other areas. This interpretation is also supported by her repeated statements that Rawls offers the strongest theory of justice that we have. All of this suggests that at least one way of reading *Frontiers of Justice* is as a supplement to *A Theory of Justice*. Viewed in this way, disability – and particularly 'mental impairment', as Nussbaum frequently calls it – figures as a special case that requires *ad hoc* solutions to an otherwise adequate notion of justice. Her general reluctance to see Rawls's reliance on Kantian personhood as founded upon the exclusion of intellectual disability downplays the problematic treatment of disability in Rawls's writings and reifies the impression that intellectual disability falls outside the scope of justice by ordinary theoretical means (see Clifford Simplican, 2015:84). Hence, as compared to my own analysis, which approaches disruptions of justice as fairness as being spaces of politicisation of the ontological underpinnings of contract thinking, Nussbaum seeks to reach closure by providing the answers that Rawls fails to deliver.

   More important than its indistinct relationship to Rawls is that there are significant internal and structural problems with the capabilities approach. An extended discussion is needed to shed light on these. Nussbaum states that her theory proposes a route to 'inclusion' for people with disabilities (2). She elaborates on two basic arguments as to why the capabilities approach performs better than justice as fairness in this regard. First, it does not ground justice in mutual advantage (156–7). Nussbaum's theory is not contractarian, which means that she does not need to postulate self-directed motivations for individuals seeking out principles governing society (158). The capabilities approach, on the contrary, starts from the reasonableness of the list of capabilities itself; it is in Nussbaum's words a theory of the good that is 'ethical all the way down' (388). As compared to procedural notions of justice, the appeal of her argument is derived from the attractiveness of the list of capabilities itself, as it lacks a metaphysical anchoring (Nussbaum, 2006:79). Hence, it may be true that, at times, individuals are motivated by mutual advantage, Nussbaum (156) states, but they are also motivated by benevolence and the love of justice itself. This means that she can rid her theory of the correspondence between those who create the contract and those who its principles apply to (15–6); the capabilities list concerns all, including those who cannot take part in formulating principles of justice or contribute to mutual advantage. This argument stems directly from Nussbaum's indebtedness to Aristotle, who famously described human beings as 'political animals'. In the capabilities approach, individuals are social creatures, naturally motivated towards others. This, in turn, provides Nussbaum with a second argument against

Rawls, challenging the rationalistic and atomistic subject he inherits from Kant. The 'political animal' gives her (2006:92) a source of human dignity outside of Kant's and Rawls's shared ideal of a rational subject: human beings are defined not only by capacities of reason but also by needs and vulnerabilities, dependence on others, and by how all of our lives are intertwined with the lives of our fellow human beings (158). Whilst Kant, as argued a few pages back, sees human dignity in the capacity to raise ourselves over our animal nature by means of reason, Nussbaum sees the split between our neediness and our rational capacities as providing dignity to human lives. Consequently, she argues that although some lives are marked by diminished reason, such lives are still worthy of our deepest respect, as they are expressions of human vulnerability and expose our shared dependency.

One way of seeing Nussbaum's list of capabilities is as expanding on a narrow focus of reason and rationality, adding dependence, emotional ties, and a social human nature as sources of human dignity. Nevertheless, she still commits to a universal understanding of what constitutes the dignified human life, and it is precisely because of this that her argument runs into problems. It is important to remember that Nussbaum's argument designates minimum requirements as concerns each capability and that these are non-interchangeable (175). According to Nussbaum – and this is a vital point for the argument that I wish to make – the minimum threshold of each capability designates the level needed to live a dignified human life (Nussbaum, 2006:70–1). Nussbaum states that beneath the threshold level 'truly human functioning is not available to citizens' (2006:71); that a life of human dignity, at least in part, is constituted by having the capabilities on the list (162); that the capabilities are fundamental for citizens (166); and that the evaluative notion of human nature operating in the capabilities approach designates normatively central aspects of humanity without which we are not living with full human dignity (179–81). As is clear from this, the notion of 'human dignity' is absolutely central to Nussbaum's conception of justice. Since each individual is regarded as an end in themselves, this means that governments are obliged to do as much as they possibly can to raise every individual to meet the thresholds levels of each capability. According to Nussbaum, the threshold levels of each capability can be specified if we imagine what a life without the capability in question would be like, a kind of mental exercise that can help establish a cross-cultural overlapping consensus concerning a minimum conception of justice (Nussbaum, 2006:161–3).

For Nussbaum's argument, all of this is important to be able to include intellectual disability: regardless of whether members of this group can be characterised as fully rational or not, all people have a claim of justice on governments in providing them with a minimum of each capability (2006:98–9). All people are subjects of justice. However, in several instances, Nussbaum states or takes for granted that (primarily intellectual) disability may have the consequence that individuals will be unable to develop all capabilities to a sufficient degree, for example when arguing that not even the best care in the world can raise all people to meet the threshold level of all capabilities (188) and that not all capabilities of people with impairment can be remedied by social action (222). She seems to think that this is especially pertinent with respect to people with what she calls 'severe mental impairments' (177; a condition not defined beyond a conceptual linkage to failing to meet Kantian standards of reason). Nussbaum's point here is that such people are still subjects of justice, as they have other capabilities for which governments have a responsibility. At the same time, these assumptions hold implications for the valuation of the inherent human dignity of such lives. As noted, Nussbaum believes that lives below the thresholds level of any capability cannot be considered fully dignified *and* that meeting threshold levels will be impossible for some. Although still subjects of justice, people who due to impairment lack any of the capabilities are not considered to be living fully dignified human lives; her inclusion of disability is paralleled with the exclusion of some people with disabilities from her conception of human dignity (see Siebers, 2010:23).

As a consequence, Nussbaum is forced to abandon her language of 'full human dignity' when speaking of people with disabilities that she presumes fall short with respect to any of the capabilities. Instead, she introduces a terminology of 'human flourishing' to specify what is attainable for people with severe disabilities (186–8). I believe that this shift of language is intentional and significant: in using the premises set up by her argument, Nussbaum is prevented from stating that people with disabilities who cannot meet all threshold levels have lives of equal human dignity – one could say that people with such disabilities disrupt her notion of the 'dignified human life' – and hence the language of 'human flourishing' is introduced as a supplement, as a new term for the state of existence that is possible in the wake of Nussbaum's simultaneous inclusion and exclusion. It shall be noted that Nussbaum (38), at one instance and only in passing, argues that she actually does grant all people born of human parents full and equal human dignity. However, this is not backed up by the actual content in her argument and is later explicitly contradicted in the discussion of people in vegetative states (who she states do not have human lives at all, regardless of their parents being human; 181–2). In summary, Nussbaum's argument of inclusion of people with disabilities excludes some people with disabilities from her notion of a dignified human life.

To be able to say something of the seriousness of the charge here, it is necessary to try to make clear what this exclusion excludes *from*: what does human dignity stand for, where does it come from, and what does it mean to not have it? To start with, this is no small matter for Nussbaum: the concept of 'dignity' is central to her notion of justice; ultimately, it is what a fair society has a responsibility to provide to its citizens. At the same time, and as Claassen (2014) notes, 'dignity' is not clearly defined in the theory. What Nussbaum says is that capabilities can be viewed as ways of realising a life of human dignity (Nussbaum, 2006:161). Capabilities and human dignity thus appear as intertwined (2011:32), and, in a sense, the capabilities list can be read as a practical operationalisation of 'human dignity'. Thus, 'dignity' is ultimately anchored in a conception of human nature or, more specifically, a conception of what it is in human beings that should be protected and nourished. For Nussbaum, 'dignity is what renders human lives noble and worthy of awe and recognition (see Gheaus, 2007; Bernardini, 2010:46).

Excluding people with 'severe' disabilities from this essentially means that we cannot be in awe of these people as human beings to the same degree as those who possess all capabilities.[5]

Revisiting the list with the arguments I have presented here in mind, it is important to remember that the capabilities have a clear functionalist slant. Thus, for example, Nussbaum (2006:77) specifies the capability of 'practical reason' by referring to its manifestations, as being able to form a conception of the good and being able to plan one's life (see Bernardini, 2010:49). This turns problematic, as the individuals of the group she seeks to reconsider as subjects of justice – people with disabilities – are defined by functional loss. It follows that unequivocal inclusion is only possible for people who do not have functional losses in what Nussbaum considers to be central capabilities. Bernardini (2010:49) has made a related point, arguing that, for Nussbaum, the inherent dignity of human beings is possible to lose – as Nussbaum herself clearly states with respect to individuals in vegetative states (181–2) – since it is something that one has by merit of capacity. In this way, human dignity is not inalienable, it is not regardless, but bound up with a set of functional characteristics. To be excluded from full human dignity thus means to be excluded from Nussbaum's humanism. This is not suggesting that Nussbaum does not value disabled lives, that she disregards them or neglects their moral significance. But it is saying that an ideal conception of human life operates in her theory as a universal yardstick, which she simultaneously assumes that some people with disabilities fail to meet. And this is a result of the fact that Nussbaum's inclusion does not question the normativity that renders people with intellectual disabilities, in particular, perpetual outsiders – it merely seeks to find a new way to care for them as part of a conception of 'justice'. It is therefore not surprising that Nussbaum – akin to what critical disability scholars have long called a 'tragedy narrative' of disability – states that the lives of people with 'severe mental impairment' are 'unfortunate' (192) and that she calls the birth of impaired children 'accidents' (102). Such formulations reveal the normative and exclusionary side of the overarching effort to include; they testify to the power of the capabilities approach to constitute certain disabled lives as worse off than 'normal'.

Reason and citizenship belonging

I have proposed two things in this chapter: (1) that the idea that 'reason' and 'rationality' are defining characteristics of humanity operates as a mechanism of exclusion in formulations of political and societal belonging and (2) that efforts to include people with intellectual disabilities that do not address this ontology will retain exclusion, resulting in situations of simultaneous inclusion/exclusion. As we shall see in the coming two chapters, the play of disruption and supplement, and hence of inclusion and exclusion, are not isolated incidents of political philosophy but permeates the politics of intellectual disability more generally. The examples analysed here are thus speaking of a more general structure inherent in liberal conceptions of subjectivity and citizenship that will manifest in intellectual disability politics circling around liberal and humanist conceptions of citizenship.

I want to conclude here by adding a few things to these propositions. First, as a reminder, it must be noted that the humanist subject was central to the ideological landscape in which 'intellectual disability' first emerged; it was in contrast with the ideals of a rational subject that 'mental deficiency' could be specified as a problem requiring government responses and scientific explanations, as I discussed in Chapter 2. Thus, the primacy of reason, exemplified by Locke, Kant, Hume, and Mill, was instrumental to the emergence of the classification of what we today call intellectual disability, and it is at present central to how liberation after state institutionalisation is figured. Hence, I have not suggested that 'liberal humanism' is disrupted because there is an inherent lack of people with intellectual disabilities, but because this branch of humanism became possible due to the exclusion of people that was perceived as lacking reason. Both the ideals of humanism and the lack of people with intellectual disabilities are socially constituted, as inside and outside, with respect to the humanist normativity.

Secondly, I want to stress again that these arguments are not meant to be read as an engagement with a number of theorists who suffer from more or less obvious prejudices against people with disability. Rather, these philosophers expose a common structure of much political thinking that I believe has become integral to how we conceive of citizenship and which is central to how we understand the deficits that define intellectual disability. Thus, in a sense, the arguments presented in this chapter illustrate Butler's (1993:xiii) proposition that any designation of a norm – in this case concerning what defines humans – will create a necessary outside of abject beings. However, the outside of reason, by being the condition of possibility for the norm itself, will always threaten the unity and homogeneity of the sphere of inclusion. The reason why deficient intelligence re-emerges throughout the history of philosophy is precisely that such threats must be put to rest, that is, that the re-emergence of disruptions provokes new supplements. Therefore, the solution to the problems here analysed will not be to seek an unproblematic inclusion of people with intellectual disabilities by continuing the search for universal grounds of societal belonging (as both Taylor and Nussbaum do). Instead, inspired by Honig (1993), I believe that precisely the disruptions caused when the sameness of citizenship confronts the difference of people with intellectual disability are resources for politicisation. When the universals, unavoidably as Butler (2005:5–6) argues, fail to include all, this very failure can serve as a starting point to critically examine the universals as such. We will continue the discussion of how critique and better possible futures of intellectual disability politics are linked in the last three chapters of the book.

Notes

1 This is also why I will not discuss related approaches, as for example the concept of 'recognition' in Honneth's thinking or the capabilities approach of Amartya Sen.
2 Today, it is widely accepted that Mill and Taylor co-authored *On Liberty*. As I follow prevailing reference standards, only Mill's name appears in references, but I want to credit both with authorship in the actual text.

3 I believe that a very similar analysis to the one advanced here could be made from Kant's political philosophy, which is strongly connected to his moral philosophy (Reiss, 1991). However, as the relationship between Kant's politics and morals is complex and continuously debated, and as his politics also is built on a social contract that is similar to Locke's (see Nussbaum, 2006:50–1), I will here focus on the subject as it appears in Kant's writing on morals.

4 Rawls is well aware that this is a simplified picture of the actual motivation of individuals. However, his argument is that benevolence and the concerns of others are served by the veil of ignorance in his theory, whilst the subjects assumed to choose the principles of justice are purposely kept one dimensional. Thus, accusations that Rawls simplifies and reduces human motivations somewhat miss their target.

5 In later discussions of 'dignity', Nussbaum (2011) argues that the potential for certain capabilities is the foundation of dignity. First, this effectively undoes her prior idea that it is 'what individuals are actually able to do' that matters for justice. Second, the problems discussed on Taylor's potentiality applies here as well; living a dignified life by merit of a capacity that one is defined as lacking hardly seems to be a convincing ascription of dignity. In *Frontiers of Justice*, however, no such admissions of potentiality are clearly made.

4 Discourse

The advent of citizenship inclusion in disability politics was both a break with and a continuation of the philosophical tradition examined in the previous chapter. In sharp contrast to a history of exclusion, governments and international organisations for the first time started to see people with intellectual disabilities as entitled to equal rights. At the same time, this was also a continuation of the liberal and humanist philosophical tradition that equates 'citizenship' with emancipation, thus re-inscribing the humanist subject as the agent to be liberated. Since intellectual disability itself is a designation of otherness to this subject – exemplified in the philosophies of Locke, Hume, and Rawls and by the history of measuring intelligence – people with this condition are both citizenship's constitutive outside and target.

In this chapter I will argue that the same structure of 'disruption' and 'supplement' that we saw at work in the history of philosophy operates in the global policy discourse: in international treatises and policies, attempts at inclusion are upset by the otherness of intellectual disability, which means that inclusion is only possible by simultaneously preserving exclusion.

This means that the global politics of intellectual disability is entrenched by two concurrent discursive constructions: first, the intellectually disabled citizen-subject is made self-ruling, independent, and worthy of inclusion. This is not the absence of power but power operating by constructing what emancipation is and what excluded subjects are expected to strive for (see Cruikshank, 1999; Rose, 1999). At the same time, exclusion lingers in the global policy discourse as the inclusion of people with intellectual disabilities is questioned, warranting exceptions or calling for special measures. This is power operating by upholding and re-inscribing otherness, post-institutionalisation. Consequently, in congruence with the conclusions of the previous chapter, the global disability discourse appears as premised on an ideal subject from which the intellectually disabled subject remains omitted. To handle this specific group, the commitment to inclusion must be supplemented by special measures, which effectively contradicts the overarching inclusive ambitions, resulting in simultaneous discourses of inclusion and exclusion.

As concerns the methods and material of what follows, the global policy constructions that will be discussed were established during the last three decades by a number of international organisations and interstate agreements committing to ideals of deinstitutionalisation, independent living, and societal participation. I will continue to call this a 'global discourse' since it is upheld by a number of international organisations that operate globally or that link their work to a cross-national political arena. However, it must be pointed out that the content of this discourse is Western in origin and linked to the humanism and Enlightenment thinking that emerged in European Modernity. I will primarily devote attention to the United Nations (UN), the World Health Organization (WHO), the European Union (EU), and the Council of Europe. Although these organisations may differ in numerous respects as concerns their respective policy commitments to disability, they share the general ideas of politics of inclusion. This also means that I will not bother with the political processes leading up to certain international policy agreements or their implementation; the focus here is how the discursive architecture of the intellectually disabled citizen-subject is constructed.

The actual material that I have worked with consists of policy documents, treatises, and agreements, primarily of the listed organisations. Reviewing this material, it is important to note that intellectual disability figures both as incorporated within the wider group of disabled people and as a sub-group specifically addressed by particular policy initiatives (see European Intellectual Disability Research Network [EIDRN], 2003:5). As concerns the UN, *the Convention on the Rights of Persons with Disabilities* (CRPD) is central. This document can be seen as an overriding framework encompassing an ideology which had come to increasingly dominate the work of various international organisations during at least the two decades before its ratification. Within the EU, the most important norm source (beside the CRPD) is the Charter of Fundamental Rights, implemented by the European Union Agency for Fundamental Rights (FRA). Hence, reports and policy statements of the FRA are important to pin down EU intellectual disability policy. Within the Council of Europe, furthermore, there has been on-going work with disability that is relevant in the context of this chapter, often related to the work of the European Court of Human Rights (ECtHR). Lastly, the work and standpoints of the WHO are most clearly summarised in their 2011 *World Report on Disability*. During the past decade, its European branch has taken a special interest in the inclusion of intellectual disability, for example seen in the *European Declaration of the Health of Children and Young People with Intellectual Disabilities and their Families*.

The chapter will proceed in two steps: first I want to pin down how the global policy discourse constructs an ideal disabled citizen-subject. Thereafter, I will show how this discourse is disrupted and hence requires supplementary amendments added to the original commitments to inclusion. As a last note of clarification, and despite the critical discussion that will follow, I recognise the important role of the CRPD, along with other international treatises and agreements, to facilitate and propagate demands that improve the living conditions of people with intellectual disabilities. My purpose here is therefore certainly not to argue for their immediate abandonment. Rather, I will examine what they might teach us about how people labelled with intellectual disability are constituted and targeted by politics.

The discursive means of inclusion

The ideas of deinstitutionalisation, self-determination, and participation emerged in the international arena during the same period as the gradual changes of national legislations and policies that brought us into the era of post-institutionalisation. In human rights frameworks, up until around 1970, disability had been largely invisible. The 1971 *Declaration on the Rights of Mentally Retarded Persons* and the 1975 *Declaration on the Rights of Disabled Persons* were both attempts to remedy this (Schulze, 2010:16). In 1993, furthermore, the UN issued the *Standard Rules on the Equalization of Opportunities for Persons with Disabilities*, which promoted equal rights and opportunities for the group (WHO, 2011:147). However, the commitments of the international community were still spread out over a considerable number of different texts, and the advent of the CRPD can be interpreted as a response to this. As such, the UN convention came to summarise a global politics of inclusion which, to some extent, was already in place. Today, the convention is frequently referred to in policy commitments of more or less all non-governmental organisations (NGOs) and international organisations. For example, the WHO world report on disability explicitly states that its purpose is to facilitate the implementation of the CRPD, and the FRA continuously refer to it in all of their recent publications on intellectual disability. Despite the fact that much of the content of the convention had been previously expressed, the CRPD is often described as signalling a shift of paradigms (Council of Europe, 2006:8; FRA, 2010), in which people with disabilities, and people with intellectual disabilities in particular, were no longer seen as unable to play an active and participating role in society. Furthermore, in addition to being a Human Rights Framework, the CRPD is designed as a development instrument that is meant to be implemented and to guide the disability politics of ratifying countries (Schulze, 2010:22).

The main idea of the CRPD is to make explicit that the universal declaration of human rights applies to people with disabilities, as well (see CRPD, Article 4; WHO, 2011:9). The necessity of clarifying this reads as an oxymoron, as the declaration of human rights would not really be universal if not already applying universally. However, in the global politics of disability, the proposed universality of such grand claims frequently comes into question when faced with certain sub-groups. In the context of the convention, the reliance on universal human rights means that its guiding principles (in Article 3) stress individual autonomy, independence, and the rights of persons with disabilities to make choices. It also commits to non-discrimination, accessibility, and respect for the differences of members of this group, and it is meant to promote their full participation and inclusion in society. Ratifying states are obliged to undertake all necessary measures to meet these ideals, including adjusting existing legislation and taking into account the situation of people with disabilities when adopting new legislations and governmental programmes (CRPD, Article 4). As concerns people with intellectual disabilities specifically, the 19th article stresses deinstitutionalisation, independent living, the right to decide where and with whom to live, along with ending all forms of segregated living.

The direction set out by the CRPD is often described in terms of the 'empowerment' of people with disabilities to control their own lives (see Council of Europe, 2006:9, WHO Europe, 2010:12) by granting access to meaningful choices (FRA, 2012:3). These descriptions hold for the general initiatives targeting all disabled people as well as the initiatives targeting those with intellectual disability specifically. An important part of this consists of 'mainstreaming' disability, which essentially means phasing out segregated services, such as sheltered employment and special education (see WHO, 2011:264). This is to be achieved by the removal of 'barriers' that are seen as hindrances to participation. The focus on barriers is especially prominent in the publications of the WHO, whose World Report is presented as a guide to remove barriers to full inclusion and thereby to implement the CRPD (WHO, 2011:xi). Thus, the WHO depicts a sphere of 'inclusion' not accessible to people with disability due to social structures and mechanisms that lock them into a corresponding sphere of exclusion. In substance, the goal is to replace segregated and institutionalising services with person-centred support, understood as a means to preserve 'dignity', to enable 'individual autonomy', and to achieve 'social inclusion' (WHO, 2011:137–8), which links back to Article 19 and 28 in the CRPD. The overarching goal of the WHO world report is that people with disabilities should be 'empowered to live in the community and participate in work and other activities, rather than be marginalized or left fully dependent on family support or social protection' (WHO, 2011:137).

As concerns intellectual disability, the European Intellectual Disability Research Network ([EIDRN] 2003:9), even before the ratification of the CRPD, had described the emergence of a new global policy direction as 'an ideological shift towards ideas of citizenship, personal control and equal access to community'. The perception of a paradigmatic shift is tightly linked to the process of deinstitutionalisation, also stressed by WHO Europe (2010:5, 2012) and the Council of Europe (2006:8, 21). WHO Europe's declaration exemplifies this line of reasoning:

> the new approach marks a paradigm shift in attitudes and approaches towards people with disabilities from viewing them as objects of charity, health care and social protection towards viewing them as subjects with rights who are capable of claiming those rights and making decisions for their lives.
>
> (WHO Europe, 2012:3)

This perception of a 'new' direction appears to be fundamental to the global disability discourse and is therefore worth having a closer look at. In this quote, like in the material more generally, the politics of inclusion becomes understandable in contrast to institutional care and paternalism. The same way as in much social scientific disability research, thus, the promotion of intellectual disability citizenship is contrasted against the repressive politics of the past (see Altermark, 2017). Drawing upon this – and throughout the material of WHO Europe, the Council of Europe, and the FRA – European states are described as being on a 'journey' towards more individualised support, where present policies have moved from seeing intellectually disabled as 'non-contributing patients' in need of care to 'citizens who need hindrances to active participation removed' (EIDRN, 2003:6). In this way 'progression' is central to the narrative of the global politics of inclusion, where the break between 'past' and 'present' constitutes a normative step forward in which old attitudes are being replaced by better ones, institutionalisation is transformed into community living, and oppression gives way to citizenship. Provided these premises, it becomes possible to describe countries that still have a substantial amount of institutional care settings as 'not having come as far', since they are supposedly on the same predestined journey towards the 'new' paradigm (see EIDRN, 2003:6). At times, the 'new' ideology of disability in this way comes close to being depicted as a historical necessity.

I argue that this narrative de-politicises present policies, which are presumed to be inherently good, in the best interests of people with disabilities, and far removed from an old paradigm of repression. As I discussed in the introductory chapter, here, power is securely placed in the past, as something we have left behind but which occasionally haunts us (see Brown, 1995:8). The references to a 'paradigmatic shift' and the existence of 'old' versus 'new' ideas elevate the ideology of the present as a set of self-evident starting points for political reasoning, un-contestable and deeply anchored in an all-embracing humanism. The prevailing problems of disability services are thereby understood as remnants of the past, and power over people with disabilities is conceived of as in the process of being replaced by individual freedom.

Closely tied to the 'present' and 'past' of disability policy is the ideal of an 'active' disabled citizen, understood in contrast to the 'passive' roles that pervaded under institutionalisation. The 'activeness' of disability citizenship is most clearly associated with 'participation'; in one's service planning, in political processes surrounding the group, in mainstream education, on the labour market, and in cultural life (see Council of Europe, 2006:12–13; WHO, 2011:137). Although the content given to these ideas tends to shift depending on which organisation we are looking at, there is an overarching discursive consensus on the value of 'activeness' rather than passivity (see Council of Europe, 2006; WHO Europe, 2010). Hence, the global discourse stipulates a citizen-subject that is integrated in society by means of working on the regular labour market, participating in mainstream education, and engaging in civil society. People with disabilities are, to a large extent, supposed to achieve this role provided the removal of 'barriers' to inclusion. Thus, the will to be active and to participate is understood to be an inherent feature for all individuals. It has been pointed out by several scholars that precisely such ideals of participation and activeness constitute a key foundation of contemporary discourses on citizenship and on democracy more generally (see McKinnon & Hampsher-Monk, 2000; Hvinden & Johansson, 2007), emerging towards the end of the 20th century and branded as an alternative to a welfare state considered too big and too clumsy that is said to make citizens 'passive' service recipients (see Rose, 1999:16–18, 141; Moriarity & Dew, 2011:684–5). Inherent to this description is precisely the insight that modes of governing shape subjectivity: an extensive welfare state that provides a high rate of coverage produces 'passive' citizens, and the task of 'activation' thus becomes to create an active and self-caring citizenry instead.

In attempting to do this, the politics of activation can be seen as integral to contemporary biopolitics. Hence, I argue that the will to be active and to partici- pate is better conceived of as an ideological construct than a given characteristic of human beings. Following Foucault's (2007) analysis of modern government, Cruikshank (1999) has argued that contemporary schemes of 'participation' and 'activation' work by a rationality of governing people by letting them govern themselves. This operates by constructing ideas of citizens as 'capable', 'inde- pendent', and 'responsible for their own good fortunes', which are, in turn, inter- nalised by citizen-subjects. Within this mode of politics, the role of the state is not to help the disenfranchised but to foster the conditions so that they can help themselves, by, for example, removing hindrances to their participation. At the same time, the power of manufacturing precisely these ideals concerning what citizenship should be is effectively veiled. Following Foucault's analysis, the global discourse of disability politics does not contain a set of evident policy goals that discard the powers that have oppressed people with disabilities but is an expression of how power operates by constructing an ideal citizen-subject that effaces its own ideology by depicting power as something primarily belonging with the repression of the past.

Parallel to the constitution of 'activeness' as an overarching ideal is the con- struction of citizen-subjects as 'independent'. To provide just a few examples: 'independence' is one of the fundamental principles guiding the Council of Europe Disability Action Plan (2006:10); the High Level Disability Group of the EU, which consists of bureaucrats from the member states, continuously refers to the importance of independence as 'choice-making'; the FRA's (2012) work on intel- lectual disability continuously emphasises this concept as a central component of quality of life; and, in the WHO world report, independence as choice making occasionally amounts to an empowered consumer role (70 1, 152–3, 158). Hence, a general feature seems to be that this concept is related to decision making, for example regarding where and how to live, how services should be implemented, and in the daily interactions between service users and public officials. This can also be linked to the previously mentioned shift in welfare politics, where the decline of extensive welfare states has been accompanied by a re-conceptualisation of the main problem of social services, from 'poverty' to 'dependency' (see Fra- ser & Gordon, 1997; Rose, 1999:159). As Verstraete (2007:58–9) points out, the frequency of descriptions of self-determination and choice as instrumental to an improved quality of life for people with disabilities is hardly surprising but reflects our present place in history, where precisely these ideals come forth as central to conceptions of what a good life entails (see Rose, 1999:87).

In summary: the move from 'past' to 'present' in disability politics is depicted as a break between 'oppression' and 'independence'. But power may not only take the form of the brute clenching of freedom that dominated the history of institu- tionalisation; it can also operate by promoting *a certain kind* of freedom, in this case as 'activation' and 'independence'. As Rose (1999:4) notes, the distinction between domination and governing is that the former attempts to crush the freedom of individuals, whilst the latter acts on it, promotes it as an overriding ideal, and utilises it for some certain purpose. This does not necessarily mean that the ideals of choice, self-determination, and independence are bad but that we fool ourselves if we approach them as transcending their social, ideological, and historical context.

Now, the ideals of the global discourse on intellectual disability policy are deeply anchored in the tradition of the humanist subject. Hence, they express the idea that people with disability shall serve for their own needs, make decisions about their own lives, and be protected from external influences while doing so. However, for this to be possible, a certain kind of subject is required, a subject that is understood as capable of making decisions, exercising self-determination, and participating in society. As was shown in the previous chapter, precisely the failure to conform to this was what provoked Locke, Hume, and Rawls to exclude people distinguished by their lack of reason from their respective notions of full societal belonging. In other words: if the biopolitics of activation and independence constitutes 'the conduct of conduct', it hinges on subjects being able to conduce in a proper way – a question which has historically and philosophically been followed by underlined question marks when it comes to people conceived of as intellectually deficient. As we shall see in what follows, these question marks persist; people with intellectual disabilities are still figured as lacking with respect to the designated yardstick of their emancipation, which means that the policy goals in question are disrupted.

Failed promises of inclusion

In the previous chapter, I discussed how groups that are seen as manifesting a lack of intelligence disrupt theorisations of citizenship. In order to handle this group, philosophical notions of societal belonging must therefore be supplemented by special measures external to its general principles. The global policies that are analysed in this chapter are themselves attempts to remedy the exclusion of people with intellectual disabilities. But as the cure is premised on the same ontology of subjectivity that caused the exclusion of the group in the first place, we here see a similar play of disruption and supplementation. We shall examine this by considering a few instances in the global policy discourse where such disruptions surface, where inclusion is withheld, and where the content of the human rights discourse is established as an ideal that cannot be met by all people with disabilities.

Inclusive education

As was noted, a key element of the global discourse on disability rights is the idea of an active and participating disabled citizen-subject. A special area of integration, continuously stressed in the material, concerns the education of people with disabilities. The Council of Europe's (2006:16) statements on the access to mainstream and integrated education illustrates the point I want to make here. Its general commitment to inclusive education reads,

> to ensure that all persons, irrespective of the nature and degree of their impairment, have equal access to education, and develop their personality, talents, creativity and their intellectual and physical abilities to their full potential.
>
> (Council of Europe, 2006:16)

Note here that the equal access to education pertains to 'all' persons, no matter the type or severity of their impairment. In line with the overriding focus on discriminatory barriers, this entails that member states actively work with legislative measures, planning, and policies to prevent segregated education. The underlying ethos is that people with disabilities should be integrated and actively participating in social life. In this context, 'equal access' translates into being provided with the same opportunities to get an education as anyone else. However, the spectre of otherness appears only a few sections later:

> in exceptional circumstances, where their professionally-assessed special education needs are not met within the mainstream education system, member states will ensure that effective alternative support measures are provided consistent with the goal of full participation.
>
> (Council of Europe, 2006:16)

Hence, there are subjects whose participation comes into question even without barriers, people who cannot be the integrated citizens that the overriding policies postulate. As seen in the previous chapter, disruptions require supplements, here consisting of the allowance of segregation which is consistent with 'full participation' due to 'exceptional circumstances'. Hence, the sphere consisting of 'all persons, irrespective of the nature and degree of their impairment' is not as inclusive as it seems; there are exceptional circumstances that break up the totality of 'all persons' and hence underhandedly constitute 'some persons' that the general principle of integrated education does not hold for. In Europe, 2.3% of all pupils are educated in segregated settings (WHO, 2011:210), and it is very likely that many or most of these have intellectual or learning disabilities, as special schooling systems often target children and adolescents with cognitive limitations more or less exclusively. It therefore seems reasonable that the 'exceptional circumstances' denote intellectual disability to a large extent.

This example is situated in a wider discussion of integrated versus segregated education (see Goodley, 2017:170–8). WHO (2011:209) states that there are two definitions of what inclusive education entails: (1) that schooling of people with disabilities should be an issue of education politics rather than of social policy and that (2) a stronger requirement of integration means that people with disabilities attend regular classes and/or have their education at the same schools as other children. If following the first definition, countries can maintain separation of people with disabilities whilst still claiming that education is 'inclusive', as long as special schooling falls under the responsibilities of the education ministry. Here, inclusion merely becomes a matter of the organisation of state administration, and it is perfectly possible to go through a whole life of such 'inclusive' education without ever setting foot in the same school buildings as non-disabled peers. The stance of the CRPD seems to conform to this view, stating precisely that inclusive education of people with disabilities requires that education authorities are responsible (see CRPD, Article 24; WHO, 2011:217). The WHO also leaves considerable room for interpretation by recommending that no new segregated schools should be built, however at the same time refusing to reproach keeping people with intellectual disabilities in separate schools. The World Report suggests, 'In practice, however, it is difficult to ensure the full inclusion of all children with disabilities, even though this is the ultimate goal' (WHO, 2011:210). Similar to the Council of Europe statements, the WHO thereby establishes an ideal that it also attaches with a clear reservation, consisting of the difficulties arising 'in practice'.

My argument here is that these ambiguities answer to the disruption of intellectual disability. The formulation of two senses of inclusive education, allowing segregated schooling to continue under 'exceptional circumstances' and the differentiation between inclusion as the 'ultimate goal' and 'in practice', are to be considered as supplements provoked by the otherness of certain people with disabilities who are seen as unable to meet the general goals of independence and integration. As education is seen to be central to inclusion, this means that the global policy discourse is tormented with lingering exclusion.

When considered on the policy level, this may not seem very upsetting; people with disabilities should be granted mainstream education, and when that is not possible, other measures directed towards the same goal shall be provided. However, what is important for my purposes is that the phenomenon of intellectual disability figures as the special case that requires extraordinary means that are external to the general goals in question. This is how the universalism of citizenship as full participation in all areas of society clashes with the particularity of cognitive deficit.

Independent living and dependency on others

I have already discussed the centrality of 'independence' of the CRPD (Article 3) and how it recurs as a reference point, for example used to specify the content of rights related to accessibility, socially integrated living, and personal mobility (Article 9, 19, 20). More generally, this is arguably a key concept of the global disability politics discourse.

Again, I want to start by looking at a specific example. In its 2006–2015 strategy, the Council of Europe (2006:10) declared that 'independence' was one of its fundamental principles, later substantiating it as 'dignity and individual autonomy including the freedom to make one's own choices'. One of the domains in which this principle has the most influence concerns where and how people with disabilities should live, which is also emphasised in Article 19 of the CRPD. On this matter, the Council of Europe (2006:20–1) action plan states,

This action line focuses on enabling people with disabilities to live as independently as possible, empowering them to make choices on how and where to live. This requires strategic policies which support the move from institutional care to community based settings.

In this quote, 'independence' has gone from being a general guiding principle to becoming a continuum that can vary in degree, as is seen in the proposition that individuals should be as independent 'as possible'. This also suggests that the guiding principle of independence cannot be fully met in all cases; otherwise the specification 'as independently as possible' would have been phrased 'to live independently' proper. The assumption that full independence is unreachable in some cases is made explicit a few sentences later:

> Full independent living may not be possible or a choice for all individuals. In exceptional cases, care in small, quality structures should be encouraged as an alternative to living in an institution.
>
> (Council of Europe, 2006:21)

The document does not specify what it means that 'full independent living' may not be a 'choice'. It seems reasonable that it relates to the 'independent living' movement of people with disabilities demanding to get appropriate support in their homes so that they can live independently. What we can infer from the quote, however, is that 'care in small, quality structures' is not seen as conforming to 'full independent living', as it is proposed as an alternative when this is impossible. Similarly to 'fully integrated education', the motivation for sidestepping the general principle is the existence of 'exceptional cases'. Considering that smaller services, such as group homes and apartments with nearby support if needed, are common among people with intellectual disabilities, it is again reasonable to assume that the 'exceptional circumstances' in question, at least to some extent, refer to people with this diagnosis. Thus, what we see here is how a general principle of 'independence' is both established and circumvented in 'exceptional cases', which means that the 'universal' principle is not really universal. An implicit division is again made within the population of people with disabilities, between individuals for whom goals of independent living are applicable and those who are characterised as 'exceptional cases' and with respect to whom these goals may be impossible to fulfil. In turn, this means that there is a need for a supplement, here appearing in the form of 'care in small, quality structures', which is a measure added outside the general envisioning of how people with disabilities should be living.

Ultimately, this relates to the dichotomy of 'independence' and 'dependence'. Consider the WHO's (2011:263) statement that reliance on institutional care, a lack of community living, and segregation are all problems that leave people with disabilities 'dependent on others and isolated from mainstream social, cultural, and political opportunities' (263). Here, 'dependent on others' is juxtaposed with the general goal of 'independence' and is clearly seen as something that contributes to the exclusion of people with disabilities. This recurring idea has implications: if 'dependence on others' contradicts 'independence', more or less all attempts to promote 'independent living' will fall short, as they leave the individual reliant on other people in granting access, removing barriers, providing quality services, and so on. Admittedly, the authors surely do not mean to imply that. What is important here, though, is not the intentions behind the wording but the structure of the relationship between 'independence' and 'dependence' that comes to the fore. In the introductory chapter, I discussed the implosion of the inside/outside structure that stems from how these poles simultaneously provide each other with meaning by merit of being opposites *and* incorporating each other; a firm and stable separation of these is impossible, as 'exclusion' will haunt 'inclusion' by being its condition of possibility. The notion of 'independence' and the efforts to formulate policies which promote this ideal can serve as examples of how this plays out. The basic logic of how 'independence' operates in the context of the policy discourse is that disabled people should become independent through the help of certain policies granting them autonomy, choice, and self-reliance. But if disabled people are to be independent only given certain policies, they are concurrently dependent on these policies to become the independent citizen-subjects prescribed. In other words, if you are independent only by being recognised as such, then your independency simultaneously reinstates your dependence on such recognition.

There is an enlightening parallel here to the peculiar double bind of summons to 'be free' (see Royle, 2003:31). When facing this particular demand, one can ignore it and hence continue to be 'un-free', as seen from the perspective of the interlocutor. If one, on the other hand, conforms to this call, one will only 'be free' by the demand of an external authority, simply obeying command, and therefore still failing to be free. Hence, when we are called upon and follow the challenge to 'be free' or to be 'independent', we are simultaneously adhering to an exterior power which either sets the terms of our freedom or incites our independence. Now, if people with intellectual disabilities were constructed as equally 'independent' as everyone else, then there would be no need for the goal in the first place, the same way that there is no need to summon people that are already 'free' to 'be free'. Paradoxically, thus, the 'dependency' that the policies aim to remove is at the same time reprised, as the intellectually disabled subject is constituted as 'dependent' on policies that prevent them from being dependent. In this way, 'independence' is perpetually haunted by its constitutive outside.

In summary, the re-conceptualisation of the intellectually disabled – from being 'dependent' to becoming 'independent' – simultaneously re-inscribes dependency at the points where the new goal is understood as unreachable. My suggestion is that this bears witness to a recurring and inherent tension between the content given to citizenship in the global policy documents and the construction of the condition of intellectual disability. As it appears, there are very few ways of understanding the present politics of intellectual disability outside these pre-set frames of interpretation; there is no language of citizenship inclusion that is able to fully incorporate its otherness.

'Full' inclusion and constitutive lack

I want to point out a final contradiction in the global policy discourse which similarly directs attention towards the structure of disruption and supplement, this time relating to the more general issue of how people with intellectual disabilities are seen as lacking with respect to what is considered a full human life.

Consider the right of citizens to vote in general elections. Of course, equality of political participation is fundamental to any contemporary conception of citizenship, and it seems contradictory to claim that individuals prohibited from voting have acquired this status. Nevertheless, this sometimes seems to be precisely the situation for people with intellectual disabilities. Full inclusion and participation in political life is central to the CRPD and integral to the work of the FRA, the WHO, and ratifying countries. At the same time, the FRA (2010:10) states that in human rights law, the right to vote is not absolute, but can be restricted, among other things, on merit of mental incapacity. In accordance, prohibition of voting rights is subjected to conditioning throughout the material. For example, the FRA states that some restriction of the right to vote can be legitimate if certain procedures and conditions are met (although it is not clear from the context of this statement whether this refers to their own position or to an established general consensus within human rights law), thereafter going on to state that it is not clear whether the CRPD prohibits restrictions of voting rights, calling for clearer guidelines on this issue (FRA, 2010:11–12). Thus, on the one hand we have a set of clearly stated commitments to equal political rights of people with disabilities and, on the other hand, a recurring suggestion that restrictions of the right to vote may be legitimate on the grounds of intellectual disability. The reason why the prohibition of voting rights on these grounds can appear to be legitimate is that intellectual disability disrupts notions of what is required for political participation. The resulting supplements consist of safeguards surrounding the retraction of their rights to vote, stating that they must be subject to careful scrutiny and should not fall on people with intellectual disabilities as a collective (FRA, 2010:10–11; WHO, 2011:171). But this is only added *after* the general goal of full and equal participation has been established. In this way, the general idea that the CRPD guarantee people with disabilities 'unconditional' human rights is haunted by the actual conditioning of certain human rights.

Another instance in which the tension between the presumed capabilities of inclusion and the construction of intellectual disability as 'otherness' surfaces is in the context of 'legal capacity', specified in Article 12 of the CRPD. The right to be recognised as a legal subject is central, since it spans different policy areas and hence affects more or less the whole life of the individual (WHO, 2010:10, 15). Ultimately, being granted equal legal standing means being seen and treated as an individual competent to make decisions in all areas of life, concerning one's living arrangements, health care, and services. To grasp what is at stake here, it is instructive to start off with a closer look at the relevant sections of the CRPD. The first three sections of the twelfth article guarantee that 'disabled people have the right to recognition everywhere as persons before the law' (UN, 2007).

Furthermore, it is assured that 'persons with disabilities enjoy legal capacity on an equal basis with others in all aspects of life'. Yet in the fourth section there is a shift of tone and focus:

> State Parties shall ensure that all measures that relate to the exercise of legal capacity provide for appropriate and effective safeguards to prevent abuse in accordance with international human rights law. Such safeguards shall ensure that measures relating to the exercise of legal capacity respect the rights, will and preferences of the person, are free of conflict of interest and undue influence, are proportional and tailored to the person's circumstances, apply for the shortest time possible and are subject to regular review by a competent, independent and impartial authority or judicial body. The safeguards shall be proportional to the degree to which such measures affect the person's rights and interests.

The quoted section deals with the rights of those who are in need of legal guardians, hence, with those who are not recognised as legal subjects after all. However, the fact that we are reading about guardianship is not made explicit in the actual text; it is an assumption that underpins the quote, a quote which would seem superfluous if the prior statement, that *all* disabled people actually were recognized as enjoying equal legal capacity and were recognised as people before the law, was really seen as unconditional. In fact, the extracted text only makes sense provided that all people are *not* recognised as having equal legal capacity.

Legal capacity and guardianship were much debated in the process leading up to the CRPD. The debate concerned whether all disabled persons could be said to have a legal capacity, and the outcome of the actual convention is often described as a manifestation of a paradigmatic shift from 'substituted' to 'supported' decision making (see Schulze, 2010:86–8; WHO, 2011:138; FRA, 2013:7). In substance, this means that individuals lacking the capacity to make choices are to be supported rather than having their decision making transferred to someone else. Both the FRA (2013:55) and WHO (2011:137–8) advocate supported decision making. Hence, in the texts analysed, the safeguards surrounding guardianship and supported decision making are juxtaposed with simply declaring some people to be legally incompetent. But by doing this, the fact that supported decision making itself is an expression of a lack of legal capacity is concealed. Thereby, the global policy discourse both upholds the idea of the universal recognition of people with disabilities as legal subjects *and* recognises that some people lack the capabilities necessary. And in this way, the shift from 'transferred' to 'supported' decision making supplements the disruption of people who fall short concerning the capacities required to be a subject before the law.

Now, this is not a legal analysis, and many of the things discussed in this chapter may well be explained in light of the intricacies of international human rights law. Neither is this a normative analysis, arguing that guardianship or supported decision making is necessarily bad. Again, the point I want to make is theoretical and concerns how intellectual disability requires that the general commitments to 'legal capacity', 'independence', and 'inclusive education' are provisionally suspended. In discourse, the construction of citizenship inclusion for people with intellectual disabilities simultaneously re-inscribes a recurring lack of capacities with respect to the ideals of citizenship. When the goals of inclusion were formulated by the disability movement, they pertained to people with disabilities in general. At the same time, the specific group of people with intellectual disabilities is understood as defined by a lack of reason, and this is why this condition repeatedly appears to be an extraordinary phenomenon that requires citizenship ideals to be added to, both in political philosophy and in policy. Hence, this condition serves as the exception which cannot be incorporated into the universalism that underpins notions of citizenship, and hence the defining incompleteness of the group comes to exist in tension with 'full' citizenship and inclusion in human rights frameworks.

Politics of inclusion/exclusion

In essence, the analysis up to this point has established two things: how a regulative ideal of citizenship is established to achieve inclusion and how this requires re-inscription of exclusion through supplements that answer to disruptions caused by intellectual disability. Hence, breaches of principles of inclusion are necessary when the idea of equality for *all* clashes with the presumed lack of reason of *some*. Furthermore, since this presumed lack of capacities is understood as a pre-political biological phenomenon, it composes a residual difference that policy can neither remedy nor incorporate. These are traces of imploding systems of signification which stretch into the organisation of services and support (as we shall see more clearly in the next chapter). The failure to include the constitutive outside establishes a situation in which 'otherness' must be both removed and reconstituted, *post*-institutionalisation. Thus, perhaps we should not be all that surprised when the ideals of independence and self-determination for people with intellectual disabilities fail to materialise, as the discourses manufacturing these ideals cannot grant citizenship without simultaneously withdrawing it.

Spivak (in Morton, 2003:28–9) has aptly captured the disciplining functions of the humanist subject by pointing out how its internalisation appears to be a precondition of becoming fully human. Considering the 'lack' that citizenship politics both answers to and reinstates, Spivak's analysis also illuminates the effect of global citizenship discourses on intellectual disability. Indeed, this group is defined as lacking in the characteristics which are commonly seen as defining humanity, made measureable by classification, and so it is to be regulated by an ideal that always seems to require its own contravention. Just as Derrida's (1997:144–6) 'supplement' highlights the incompleteness of the linguistic sign, 'intellectual disability' highlights the incompleteness of discourses of 'citizenship inclusion'. This, again, points to why this particular kind of disability is central to understand citizenship and inclusion in general. In a way, what has been analysed here is the failure to reach closure, the failure to integrate otherness, precisely because such integration threatens the system of signification that citizenship is founded upon in the first place. Including the constitutive outside of what creates our sense of 'normal' subjectivity also means putting the very normality of this subjectivity into question. In this way, the policy promises made on a discursive level are always already broken; the failure to include, often noted and criticised by disability scholarship as an anomaly, should rather be approached as a feature of a system which can already be detected when examining how the goals of inclusion are given their discursive shape. This is not to say that citizenship politics is not called for or that it just constitutes more of the same in relation to institutional care. Rather, it is to say that we are mistaken when suggesting that citizenship discourse is unequivocally inclusive. Now, in the next chapter, we will see how this structure – of simultaneously crafting intellectually disabled citizen-subjects and excluding them from citizenship – transforms into technologies of government applied in services where this kind of citizen-subject is supposed to materialise.

5 Control

In this chapter, I will show how disability services both foster citizenship and enforce constraints on citizenship rights. Hence, contrary to the standard interpretation, the emergence of politics of inclusion did not simply move power from state representatives to disabled individuals; it transformed how power governs the individuals targeted. On the one hand, in disability services, power has come to operate by moulding citizens and manufacturing ideals of self-determination, participation, and independence. On the other hand, individuals with intellectual disability are recurrently subjected to paternalism and enforcements in case their behaviour does not conform to the ideals of citizenship. Both of these are effectuated through specific techniques and routines of support workers in their everyday work. Together, the dual logics of manufacturing and restricting citizenship define the service provision of post-institutionalisation.

To start with: in most social scientific and philosophical studies of this concept, 'citizenship' is usually linked to equality of civil, political, and social rights, conceptualising it as a *status* (Marshall, 1950). On the contrary, my analysis starts from the proposition that this notion produces subjects (see Cruikshank, 1999). Hence, 'citizenship' will be understood as an institutionalised discourse that establishes ideals for the relationship between the individual, the state, and the community, shaping how people come to relate to the societies that they live in (see Yuval-Davis, 2007). Therefore, while the standard narrative of disability politics primarily understands power as an intrusion on citizenship, I will analyse how power operates by shaping how individuals aspire to become and how they understand themselves as 'citizens' (see Cruikshank, 1999).

As was stressed in the introductory chapter, disability services that are supposed to promote inclusion have often failed to meet the ambitions of policy commitments to citizenship inclusion. Thus, the overriding conclusion of Beadle-Brown et al. (2007 in Clement & Bigby, 2010), that deinstitutionalisation is ridden with remnants of the institutional era that constrain the possibility of independence and self-determination, seems to capture a global tendency in residential and community care for people labelled with intellectual disability (see Galvin, 2004). Still, as I discussed in the introduction, the standard interpretations of the situation are blunt and misrepresent the problems: rather than implementation failures or remnants of institutionalisation, I will argue that we are dealing with a new regime of government that is defined by the simultaneity of inclusion *and* exclusion.

I will build this argument by showing that two concurrent rationalities under-pin actual work in intellectual disability services. Both of these are integral to the present biopolitical regime. First, service provision operates by 'governmen-tality' (Foucault, 2007:107–10, 115–23), a mode of government geared to cre-ate self-ruling subjects by nurturing capacities seen as necessary to function as a citizen. This is not power that restrains freedom but that incites people to be free in a particular way. At the same time, service provision operates by the use of technologies of discipline, restriction, and straightforward coercion, which con-strain the freedoms associated with citizenship (see Foucault, 1991). Together, these parallel modes of government create a decentralised system of control, con-stantly monitoring whether people with intellectual disabilities are fit to make judgements regarding their own lives. Furthermore, and as we shall see, this new regime of government operates in and through relationships formed at the lowest levels of policy implementation, between support workers and people with intel-lectual disabilities living in group homes.

A few words need to be said about the methodological considerations that have guided this specific chapter. In essence, this is a case study of Swedish intellec-tual disability services. There are strategic reasons to pinpoint Sweden in order to grasp the politics of inclusion. As stated already, for the past 30 years poli-cies targeting individuals with intellectual disabilities have undergone significant shifts in large parts of Europe and North America, from institutional confinement to policies focusing on citizenship and socially integrated living. In this context, the Swedish legislation, called the Law of Support and Service for Certain People with Disabilities (LSS), can be seen as a forerunner (see Hollander, 1999:409–10; Race, 2007:32). More generally, Sweden is renowned in the international disabil-ity community for its ambitious goals of societal integration and its strong focus on individual self-determination (see Kristiansen, 1999; Kristiansen et al., 1999; EIDRN, 2003:5–9, 51–60; Race, 2007:23–5, WHO, 2011:148, 156). Therefore, Sweden is an exemplary case to theorise the government of intellectual disability after deinstitutionalisation.

I will draw on two sources of material: official documents and evaluations of intellectual disability services and interviews with support workers and activists diagnosed with intellectual disability. The interview material is made up of 33 interviews with support workers and bureaucrats, whereof 26 are with staff work-ing at the street level, in direct contact with people with intellectual disabilities, and the rest with first-line managers and bureaucrats. Swedish disability policy is primarily implemented on the municipal level, and 17 of the interviews were conducted as a case study of one such large Swedish municipality, and a second set of 13 interviews was conducted in three other municipalities. Since the con-clusions that will be presented appear to hold over time and across municipal borders, there is no need to differentiate between the initial case study and the follow-ups in the actual text. In addition, I have interviewed five members of the self-advocacy organisation Grunden who have first-hand experience of Swed-ish disability services in several different municipalities. This took the form of a group interview (which will be more thoroughly presented in Chapter 7). Finally, the focus has been on one specific service, namely supported living, which is most often organised as group-home living or as satellite apartments (we will get back to what this means in a moment). The group home is the most common form of accommodation in the wake of deinstitutionalisation, in Sweden and elsewhere, being singled out by Tøssebro (2005) as the emblematic form of integrated community living. Hence, it is a good place to start looking for how power operates after deinstitutionalisation.

The citizen-subject of Swedish disability politics

The politics of inclusion of Sweden is associated with two significant legislative changes: the Omsorgslag ('the Care law') of 1985, characterised by its focus on citizenship and self-determination and the introduction of the LSS in 1994, which replaced the Care law and established disability services as rights. The LSS strengthened the idea of citizenship as encompassing 'independence', 'self-determination', and 'societal integration' and was warmly welcomed by the disability movement as well as by all parties in the Swedish Parliament. A direct result of the new law was that the remaining institutions were closed down and replaced by socially integrated living, meaning that Sweden became one of the first countries to deinstitutionalise disability support (Tideman, 2005; WHO, 2011:147). In the narrative of Swedish disability politics, the LSS marks a shift of paradigms in which people with intellectual disabilities were finally recognised as equal citizens. Although Swedish policy has undergone several changes since the emergence of the LSS, the direction set out by the 1994 reform has been maintained.[1]

The LSS states that public services for people with intellectual disabilities aim to make the targeted individuals independent and participating members of society (7 § LSS; Prop. 1992/93:159), and the law is structured around 10 services which are designed to accomplish this (9 § LSS). Supported living, which will be the main focus here, is, for example, accompanied by sheltered employment and personal assistance.[2] Furthermore, LSS is a law of rights, which means that individuals deemed to be in need of support and who have a diagnosis which makes them eligible have a legal claim that the municipality of residence provide them with services. The overall ambition of the 'handicap reform' in 1994 was to move power from the state to individuals with disabilities (see Grassman et al., 2009:45). An important means to achieve this movement can be found in the strong emphasis on protecting the 'self-determination' and 'autonomy' of individuals with disabilities (6 § LSS). These formulations must be understood against the backdrop of paternalistic institutional confinement, which was depicted as the main problem throughout the public commissions that led up to the 1994 reform (SOU, 1990:19; SOU, 1991:46; SOU, 1992:52). Along these lines, Swedish disability politics is designed to establish a sphere of individual integrity and autonomy that is protected against state intrusions and paternalism of the kind that was commonplace during the 20th century. As such, the politics of inclusion, and the LSS more specifically, are tightly connected to the main tenets of the liberal and humanist conceptions of citizenship; by their emphasis on rights, by the perceived conflict between state and individual, and by the weight given to 'self-determination' and 'independence' as central goals.

In summary, thus, Swedish policy bears the hallmarks of the politics of inclusion. As we shall see in what follows, also here, the ideals of citizenship comes into friction with understandings of intellectual disability, which means that we shall see a similar play of disruption and supplement as in the previous two chapters.

Making and failing citizens

First, a few essential notes about the empirical context. The nature of work in supported living can look very different, for example between group homes and satellite apartments (apartments where individuals do not have access to constant support and which are most often integrated into regular housing estates), between different group homes, but also between individuals living at the same group home. Some individuals only need help with structuring their daily routines while getting by independently in most other respects. Others need help with personal hygiene, eating, dressing themselves, and leaving the home. Despite such differences, the goals of self-determination and participation in society apply, although the legislation states that these goals should be interpreted with respect to the needs of the individual (2 § LSS). Among the support workers I have interviewed, the whole range of service needs and severity of disability is covered.

In the typical Swedish group home – the dominant way of organising supported living – five to seven apartments are bundled together along with larger rooms that are shared between all tenants.[3] Sometimes, staff is also responsible for one or a few satellite apartments where people with less time-consuming support needs live. The personnel in group homes usually have a high school degree, and there are commonly about six to eight regular staffers working in each group home. It is a low-paid job considered to have low status. Group homes are usually located in either suburban residential areas of self-contained houses, where the group home is often visibly separated from other houses in the neighbourhood, or in regular housing estates. Many people with intellectual disabilities spend a large part of their life within the confines of the group home, perhaps going to sheltered employment centres for work and leaving for daytrips together with other tenants during the weekends. But there are of course also individuals who go out on their own and have friends, activities, and so on.

In the following, we shall start by seeing how support workers actively strive to cultivate citizens. Thereafter, we shall consider the concurrent technologies of constraining the freedom and independence of people with intellectual disabilities.

Producing citizens

The purpose here is to produce a detailed understanding of what the politics of inclusion means in the actual contexts in which it meets people with intellectual disabilities. To start with: all of the interviewees express that they value the general intention of the LSS to enable people with disabilities to live independently and by their own choices. The commitment to the goals of 'independence', 'participation', and 'self-determination', however, far from implies that the interviewees are neutral with respect to how the people they work with live. To the contrary, they continuously seek to encourage certain ways of being, develop certain capacities, and teach certain lessons on how to get by in society. It is clear that the people interviewed see it as their task to facilitate the individuals they work with to *become* citizens. Furthermore, as has been discussed with reference to the history of political philosophy and policy discourse, citizenship is frequently described as premised on certain capacities that are actively nurtured and promoted; one needs to be able to make choices, to move around society, and to reflect on the consequences of one's actions. Much of what goes on in the group home is geared towards creating such individuals, capable of being independent. This focus is often already evident when the interviewees answer a first general question about the overriding purpose of their work:

> The whole point of our workplace is to make the people living here as able to participate as possible. They cannot be totally independent, but to make them as able to participate as possible in different decisions concerning their lives.
>
> (AP7)

> The idea is to make them more independent. So I work to make myself redundant. You want as little support for them as possible. But, they live here for a reason, so it's not possible to make them accomplish what people such as you and I can do. But you can make them less dependent on support.
>
> (CP1)

Depending on the service needs of the individuals one works with, 'independence' might mean being able to choose what to eat or getting the newspaper out of the post-box, whilst for other individuals, it could mean being able to walk to and from the sheltered employment centre or being able to go out and eat on one's own at a restaurant. It is continuously stressed that such development is a process, in which tenants in the group home gradually learn how to manage their lives.

Taken together, the interviews establish the impression that the laws and regulations of Swedish disability politics incite processes of shaping individuals to become citizens. One of the interviewees describes this:

> It's both them and us that see the need for developing skills. We talk to them and ask 'would you like to do this?', for example. And then we'll have to wait and see what the response is. Sometimes, you have to ask and ask and ask and ask, for three months, ask and ask and then ask again, before they are ready. Then, we discuss how to do it, how they can learn. So that discussion is always there, these are really long processes.
>
> (CP3)

The quote is typical in how it describes staffers as initiators and highly active in nurturing capacities. In several interviews, the processes of developing skills of independence and participation are described as developing through carefully managed progression, where staff teaches individuals with intellectual disability how to improve skills understood as required to be participating and self-determined community members. One of the support workers gives an example of this:

> One of the persons living here could not walk by herself to her day-care centre, despite it being just a kilometre away. Her parents said that she had to take the taxi. But we decided that we would work with her, so we started to walk with her, gradually letting her walk more of the way by herself. We planned, step by step, how she could learn how to walk to and from work.
>
> (CP4)

This quote illustrates the general tendency that people with intellectual disabilities are not seen as already possessing the necessary capabilities of citizenship. This picture is mirrored in previous research on the implementation of citizenship politics in other countries. Consider, for example, the description provided by Gilbert (2003:40) of how self-management and citizenship are actively promoted and developed by the UK public officials he interviews. Similarly, Schelly (2008), describes the actual experience of working as a personal assistant implementing policies of self-determination as a process of cultivating capacities. In these accounts, making one's own decisions, taking responsibility, and communicating one's desires are skills that are taught rather than capacities that people with intellectual disabilities have. Rather than 'empowerment', this can be seen as a reinforcement and practical application of what Clifford Simplican calls the 'capacity contract': processes aiming to instil in the individual the prerequisites of societal belonging, echoing what Cruikshank (1999) calls processes of crafting 'citizen-subjects'.

Since developing skill sets necessary for citizenship is seen as integral to working at the group home, there is a need to coordinate and plan how these processes are managed. A common way of doing this is to discuss tenants at monthly staff meetings. These are more or less ubiquitous in group homes and are very often devoted to discussing how the development and behaviour of each individual should be handled. A related tool to coordinate citizen production is the report book, where what has happened during the day (or night) is written down. These often function as logs of activities, visits, and similar – but sometimes they also map the moods of tenants, whether they have requested certain things, whether they have demanded help with certain tasks, or whether they have showered, brushed their teeth, or eaten. The report book appears to be central to the working routines of supported living, keeping track of matters such as personal hygiene, mental states, or when and for which reason tenants have left their apartments. The activists of Grunden share the impression that report books are central to the organisation of supported living; they are well aware that they are being reported about and are talking points at meetings in their absence, which they describe as derogatory. One of the activists recalls how she contested such practices, demanding to see what was reported about her and to be present when talked about, but these requests were denied by staff. As described in my conversation with Grunden, in these cases, the efforts to plan and coordinate measures to produce citizens could not extend to involve the citizens-to-be in the process.

Far from a withdrawal of state representatives, thus, the nurturing of citizenship functions by planned and coordinated processes where staffers see it as their role to cultivate capacities which are understood as being necessary for citizenship. A recurring theme here concerns capabilities of decision making. There is a widespread idea among the support workers that people diagnosed with intellectual disability have difficulties making choices, which becomes problematic considering the weight of self-determination and independence in the LSS. Basically, this is the disruption of 'intellectual disability' to conceptions of reason as a qualification for citizenship that I have discussed in the previous two chapters. It shall be noted that the perceived lack on behalf of individuals granted support is not described as pertaining to making choices in general but to making 'good' choices. However, since the interviewees interpret the LSS as a hindrance against making decisions on behalf of the individuals they work with, they often set out to shape the decision making of tenants in ways that do not violate their interpretation of the law. In this context, all interviewees state that 'motivational work' is central to their jobs. The selection of quotes that follows illustrates what this can mean:

> All we can do is to work through motivating. It is the same problem as with what they eat, for example. If they want to eat kebab seven days a week, then we are not allowed to force them not to.
>
> (BP2)

> Very much depends on the individual. We have people living here with mild disabilities, many of which have gone to regular schools and have a good understanding of things . . . with them it is continuous motivational work, where they have a very clear awareness of their rights. With young people, there is a lot of motivational work. People with more severe disabilities are not aware of their rights in the same way, although relatives might be. But that cannot mean that you just ignore their wishes. After all, it's always about motivation.
>
> (AP6)

> I believe that respect for the individual is central, that you try to avoid infringements. You have to use your common sense. If they want to sleep 'til 1 p.m. we cannot stop them, and then they'll sleep 'til 1 p.m. We have to motivate them against doing these things if we believe that they're not good for them.
>
> (AP10)

As it appears, motivation occurs when there is a conflict between what support workers and individuals living in group homes believe is best in a certain situation. Thus, the 'lacking' decision-making capacity which is referred to essentially consists of not agreeing with the judgement of support workers, indicating that the interviewees presume that their own viewpoint is superior. In this way, motivation functions by directly intervening in the individual's field of action not by constraining or forcing but by seeking to convince and win over. The technology is applied to choices concerning a number of different things, such as what clothes to wear, what to eat, how to use one's money, how many cups of coffee to drink, or less mundane matters such as how to handle a relationship or what assistance tools to use. There are also great differences concerning how 'motivation' is carried out:

> Some people, we can talk to. One person here, if she had been investigated today, she would probably not have ended up in the LSS. You can joke with her. So, with her, you can say 'you won't feel well if we go there, let's do something else instead'. There is another person here where it's much harder [when he wants to go somewhere that makes him feel ill]. I have tried to explain to him that 'you are older now, you don't think that it is comfortable to go there . . . Shouldn't we stay home and have coffee and cookies instead?' You only have sweets and biscuits to use, that's what's left if they cannot use their hands.
>
> (AP4)

> You constantly need to guide them in their self-determination and decisions. It is about informing and pointing out why certain things are important [to think about when choosing]. Sometimes, it is not possible, but oftentimes you can argue with them. It is never about forcing, because we are not allowed to do that.
>
> (AP10)

> If you're accompanying them buying clothes, then you have to steer a little and say 'don't you think this shirt is nicer?' On the other hand, you have to step back if they insist. We have a man living here who does not want to clean up his room, so we have to go in to him. But he can still say that we have to leave, and in that case, we have to. So you often think 'should he just sit there in his mess?' But if someone came in and told me to go somewhere or do something, I would become really pissed off.
>
> (AP1)

Thus, motivation can entail verbal persuasion, elaborate arguing, providing information, reminding of consequences, bribing with sweets, and making suggestions, among other things. Many interviewees stress that verbal communication is their primary working tool, especially when it comes to motivational work. It is common that support workers describe elaborate discursive techniques that make certain choices appear to be more favourable and attractive, as is exemplified in the question 'Don't you think this shirt looks nicer?' In several interviews, it is also stressed that tenants with intellectual disability view the support workers as authorities. Thus, prior to motivation is a hierarchical relationship, which suggests that we are not dealing with regular advice giving like you would find in most relationships between friends or siblings. Motivation is not presented as input into the decision-making process of people with intellectual disabilities but as a measure that seeks to produce the *correct* decisions.

Motivational work is also described in my conversation with the activists of Grunden, who see it as a recurring annoyance in their everyday lives. All of them have stories about being 'advised' and, as they see it, protected from negative consequences, for example regarding not having their partners staying overnight, not being out too late, and not drinking alcohol. The extent and frequency of references to 'motivation' in the material presents it as an ever-present dimension of how people with intellectual disabilities are communicated with by group home staffers. Thus, motivation is a technology of micro-scale management that can be seen as arriving both *before* and *after* citizenship: on the one hand, it is a response to citizenship, to the perceived gap between the rights of freedom and the perceived incapacity to make wise use of it. On the other hand, considering the extent and ubiquitous nature of its use, it must also be seen as a continuing project of crafting citizen-subjects, shaping individuals to be able to act as good decision makers. As such, motivation supplements the disruption caused by people with intellectual disabilities and their incapacity for making good decisions.

As a technology of power, motivation arises in the context of post-institutionalisation, when collectivism and rules give way to individualism and freedom of choice. This is aptly captured in the following quote:

When we started with individualised meals and they were allowed to decide what to have, they gained weight, of course. But I am not allowed to say 'no'. I am allowed to explain that it isn't good to have pizza seven days a week. But if she still wants it, then I am in no position to decide over them. So, we try, like, saying that 'you had pizza the other day, wouldn't it be nice with a salad?'

(CP3)

This illustrates how the abandonment of collective rules and restrictions produces a new set of perceived problems facing support workers. Motivation arises in this context as a technology applied to manage tenant behaviour in situations in which the freedom of the individual risks leading to bad decisions. This is power transformed, from collectively enforced rules to individual management. For example, to restrict 'bad' eating habits, motivation works by seeking to convince each individual of the consequences of being overweight, of the dangers of diabetes, and so on. In turn, the lives of individuals become embedded in these discourses, constituting a landscape in which considerations of health effects of eating habits become incorporated into how people with intellectual disabilities practice their right to live by self-determination. This corresponds to Foucault's notion of government as the 'conduct of conduct'; instead of deciding what people with intellectual disabilities eat, the management of the individual seeks to make its targets internalise health considerations into their individual decisions – that is, to achieve a subject that conduces in the favoured way.

Two features of the technology of motivation stand out. First, motivational work always takes the individual as its target, and it is described as requiring a deep knowledge and bond of commitment between tenant and staffer. Second, motivational work presumes a hierarchy, where the support worker doing the motivating perceives their own viewpoint as superior. Otherwise, motivation would not be needed and could not be justified. For the motivation to function efficiently, furthermore, it is necessary that the recipient of motivation also perceives the knowledge of support workers as authoritative. Otherwise, they will not listen. In one of the group homes where I conducted interviews, the hierarchy of knowledge regarding decision making was made explicit:

> Here, we work with providing them with 'good' and 'bad' choices, where we explain that if you do this, it will have bad consequences, but if you do that, you will gain from it long term. If you choose the bad course of action, then you have to live with the consequences. It is not about punishing them, but about building on what's positive.
>
> (CP3)

This way of working amounts to redesigning the field of action, attaching a discourse of valuation to courses of action. Like motivational work more generally, this is described as a tool to increase and allow for self-determination, as the individual remains in control of whether the 'good' or 'bad' alternative is chosen. Of course, in all motivational work, such valuation is implied by the fact that motivation is seen as required and possible to justify. What happens when courses of action are explicitly named this way is that the otherwise taken-for-granted authority of knowing what is best is made explicit.

In conclusion, the reality of group home work ties well into what Rose (1993:285) has deemed a prominent feature of contemporary government, namely the decentralised management of the choices of individual citizens. The technologies of citizen-production described here, furthermore, reveal that such micro-management occurs no matter the severity of disability: nurturing capacities may mean teaching individuals how to post a letter or how to develop information-gathering skills in preparation for the general election, depending on the individual targeted. In this way, implementing the goals of the LSS, designed to foster independence and self-determination, paradoxically appears as an intensification of state involvement in the lives of people with intellectual disabilities. This is a transformation of the relationship between the state and the individual, where government no longer confronts people with intellectual disabilities as a collective, denied rights and subjected to paternal decision making, but constantly manages and promotes the capacity of individuals to become self-ruling. The power inherent to such shaping is blatantly obvious to the activists of Grunden, as it permeates their everyday lives. They tell me about constant tensions with staff, about recurring reminders, advices, and a sense of being controlled and watched over.

In this way, the politics of post-institutionalisation is characterised by management of the individual, guided by how support workers interpret the LSS and what capabilities they perceive as necessary to function as a citizen. However, this is not necessarily meant to imply that this way of working cannot be justified. One may well argue that technologies of motivation are necessary and good for the individual. Rather, my point is that we fool ourselves if we do not see them as instances of power. Like in Foucault's analysis, we need to disentangle questions of power from normative judgements; in order to have informed conversations regarding whether the technologies I have described here are worthwhile – discussions that need to involve people with disabilities being granted these services – we need to arrive at an appropriate understanding of what they are. Now, in the following, we shall see how post-institutionalisation is characterised by another type of supplement, in which the discrepancy between citizenship ideals and intellectual disability instead give rise to restrictions that clearly violate the legislation and its ethos of inclusion.

Failed citizens

A common rhetorical figure, reappearing in more or less all contexts in which LSS services are managed, is that people with intellectual disabilities 'after all are living here for a reason'. This figure of expression usually accompanies the idea that the LSS cannot be adhered to at all times and indicates that there are characteristics of intellectual disability which conflict with the idea of citizenship. A number of my questions encourage the interviewees to put into words what they feel is difficult with respect to the LSS. The answers suggest that there is a widespread perception of a conflict between the right of self-determination and the very reason why people with intellectual disabilities are entitled to support, namely their intellectual deficiencies. Like in the history of political philosophy and the global discourse of citizenship inclusion, there is a will to include what is perceived as impossible to fully realise. All but a few support workers explicitly state that people with intellectual disabilities sometimes do not know what is best for them, which means that the self-determination of members of this group is being called into question:

> They cannot see the consequences of their actions. Sometimes, self-determination is not what is best for them. Within LSS, there are not many that can do that. So in the end, you often end up with how the staff view things, I don't think that can be avoided. You try to do what is best for the person in question.
>
> (AP4)

> In pure intellectual terms, they are at the level of minors. That's how it is. Although they are formally viewed as adults.
>
> (CP1)

> Conflicts between what's best for them and what they want are very much a part of our daily work. They don't have full capacity, that's why they live

here. And I think that they should have a right to being cared for, rather than decide everything. They cannot be responsible for all their choices and that's when things turn strange with a law stating that they have a very strong right for self-determination.

(BP2)

As exemplified in these quotes, the lack of ability ascribed to people with intellectual disabilities is seen as inherent to why these people need support in the first place; 'they live here for a reason', and that reason is the deficiencies that serve as the basis of their diagnosis. This is not unique to the Swedish context. For example, in his study of the UK, Gilbert (2003:40) has pointed towards a widespread lack of belief in the capabilities of people with intellectual disabilities. In effect, this suggests that individuals with intellectual disability are not only understood to be 'citizens in the making' but also 'failed citizens', unable to exercise all of the rights granted by politics of citizenship because of their impairment (see Clement & Bigby, 2010:128). Consequently, many care workers express an overt frustration with the focus on self-determination and individual choice of the legislation:

I have no education, so I have never read the complete law. But I have been informed about it. And I do feel constrained. Many times, I have been in conflict with the LSS when I have felt that things I have done have violated the law. But if I had not acted as I did, it would have been wrong. It does feel awful, really, it sure does. [. . .] But, sometimes it is right to violate the law. Hopefully people have enough sense to see what's wrong and right.

(AP1)

It sounds really nice that everyone should be participating and equal, but it does not work . . . They . . . [the formal rules] destroy much more than they heal. Sometimes when I get home, I want to vomit on all of these laws and regulations.

(AP8)

They cannot see consequences but we are really not allowed to do anything until it is a life threatening situation. It is really upsetting that you can only look . . . after all, you are a fellow human as well.

(BP1)

Similar frustrations are described in research of other national disability support systems as well. Consider for example Clement and Bigby's (2010:98, 128) description of how UK care workers argue that the goal of autonomy and independence 'does not take disability into account' since it ignores the lacking intellectual capacities of the targeted group. Implicit here, and throughout my interviews, is precisely that goals of autonomy and independence are premised on capacities of reason and rationality that individuals with intellectual disability allegedly lack. In my material, furthermore, such sentiments are also expressed by staffers who make overarching statements of commitment to politics of inclusion.

The perception that disability is not taken into account by policies protecting self-determination and independence easily slips into a paternalistic style of reasoning:

> You try to work with as much self-determination as possible. But I can say as much, the guy that I take care of, if we are out buying clothes, we buy what I like. Otherwise, he would look really strange and, I mean, you don't have to make them stand out even more. Beanies in particular, for this poor guy . . . there probably is not a thing to put on that head that he looks good in. You don't have to make it wackier than it already is.
>
> (AP4)

Under the previous heading, a similar situation spurred another interviewee to motivate the individual. Here, this staffer rather describes herself as an 'intervener'. This kind of steering, deciding over and forcing, reoccurs in the material with respect to very different kinds of situations:

> According to the law, they are allowed to decide everything. You think a lot about that in certain situations. Sometimes it feels as if they do not know what is best for them. So you have to step in a little. We have a person living here that prefers to stay inside, all the time, but if she does come out she is really happy. But she can't see that while inside. So sometimes you just say to her 'now, put on your shoes so we can take a walk'. But I am not allowed to do that. I have to ask. But if I ask she says 'no'. Still, when she is out, she is so happy, while inside she has outbursts and gets angry. So in such situations, I do the wrong thing, but is it really wrong to make her happy?
>
> (AP1)

> If some people want to eat ice cream all the time, then you have to steer them. I mean, you see that all the time with your own kids at home, they are not allowed to eat candy and sweets all day. Myself, I might prefer to have chips instead of sausages with mashed potatoes, but I have an insight that this is not good for me.
>
> (AP8)

> Steering is ever-present and can be about something like care-workers believing that it's silly that Muslims don't eat pork. That has happened, a care worker serving pork to an unaware disabled Muslim woman. That is just one example of where personnel and tenants can have completely different views.
>
> (AP12)

The second quote is particularly interesting in this context, since it highlights how non-disabled individuals, like the interviewee herself, also make poor choices.

Indeed, people without disabilities can smoke a lot of cigarettes, drink a lot of alcohol, be really overweight, get diabetes as a result, and numerous other things that disabled people are described as being prevented from doing. The difference is that non-disabled individuals are depicted as acting against their better judgement, whilst people with intellectual disabilities, in these situations, are described as being incapable of incorporating consequences into their deliberations on how to act. There is a presupposed difference of sorts between the presumably oblivious behaviours of people with intellectual disabilities and the harmful actions against better judgement of non-disabled people. This leads to the paradox that ideas of normality become more restrictive for people with disabilities than for the non-disabled; people with this diagnosis are not allowed to wear beanies that make them stand out, to pick an example from the earlier quotes, even though people without this condition wear them. The difference is that individuals without this label supposedly know that they look silly, whilst people with intellectual disabilities are seen as lacking this self-reflexive capacity. Similarly, in many group homes, there are restrictions concerning how many cups of coffee tenants are allowed to have, what days they are permitted to eat sweets, what kinds of stuff they are allowed to spend their money on – all in clear conflict with the ethos of Swedish disability policy and all legitimised by an idea of normal living that is narrower and much more carefully guarded for this group than it is for the general population (see Yates et al., 2008:249).

Thus, the perception of people with intellectual disabilities as being unable to see the consequences of their actions not only incites motivational work but can also provide support workers with a justification for deciding over the people they work with. In these situations, the ethos of citizenship is supplemented by technologies that are seen as breaching the law. This way of justifying restrictions and coercion is brought up in a clear majority of the interviews and in all municipalities that I have visited.[4] This is also mirrored in the conversations with the members of Grunden, who indicate that experiencing restrictions and having their rights to self-determination and autonomy curtailed are commonplace, not only for them personally but also for the members of their organisation in general. Their stories can be seen as depicting the LSS as in a continuous state of exception, where support workers can decide when the rights of independence and self-determination should be departed from. In their view, this has severe and devastating consequences for people with intellectual disabilities, as the paternalism of present disability services crushes self-confidence, hurts people's independence, and produces a lot of suffering.

Although infringements on decision making can occur in almost any conceivable situation in the supported-living setting, there are some kinds of situations that recur in the material and that I want to mention here. The first one concerns what people with intellectual disabilities are allowed to eat. Interestingly, when asked open-ended questions about whether the interviewees know of situations in which restrictions are employed or can be justified, they often spontaneously give eating habits as an example. The efforts that go into achieving good eating habits are also stressed by the members of Grunden, which asked why healthy food should be such an overt concern for people with intellectual disabilities whilst the staffers are allowed to eat whatever they want. In several group homes that I have visited, dinner is eaten collectively, and food is ordered from a supplier that the municipality has an agreement with. At these places, staff decides what is served and do the cooking, although possibly allowing tenants to put in a request for their favourite dish once a week. A more drastic measure to this end, which has been described to me as occurring in several different municipalities, is to put padlocks on the refrigerators of tenants: people with intellectual disabilities are allowed to buy whatever they like as long as they agree that the food will be locked up.

A second area in which restrictions seem to be frequent revolves around sexuality. A first-line manager (AM4) told me that she found out that the tenants of a group home that she managed were given birth control pills without consent. Outside of the formal interviews, several bureaucrats have told me that this occurs in other municipalities as well. Although the scope of such practices also requires a more systematic examination, their very existence is both worrying and analytically important. When speaking with the activists of Grunden, they share similar experiences. One of them describes how she was told by staff that she would only be allowed to live in a satellite apartment if she agreed to insert a birth control hormone stick. Another member recounts how she was not allowed to have guests of the opposite sex stay overnight and a third that she was frequently visited by staff when she had her boyfriend over, which she perceived as a poorly masked attempt to monitor what they were doing.

Lastly, a third restriction of the formal goals of the politics of inclusion concerns the freedom of movement. This is sometimes manifest just by looking at how supported living is built. For example, I know of several group homes surrounded by locked gates. The activists in Grunden state that locked doors are commonplace in order to ensure that tenants do not leave without the permission of staff. They also tell me how staffers often demand to know where they are going when leaving and require that they be home at certain times. Similar stories are shared by first-line managers. This presents itself as a form of *de facto* confinement, in direct conflict with the Swedish constitution (8 § RF, 2 kap.). These restrictions of when and how people with intellectual disabilities are allowed to leave their homes blatantly contradict any common conception of citizenship.[5]

To summarise: the productive power of 'governmentality' targets individuals presumed to be capable of acting rationally and intentionally. Since people with intellectual disabilities are understood as at least partly lacking these capabilities, there is a need to complement this technology of subject formation with discipline and coercion. In this way, supported living is characterised by actively producing citizens that are included whilst also targeting them with technologies of exclusion (see Gilbert, 2003:40). And so people with intellectual disabilities remain Others, even within the services that should be advocating for their inclusion. As before, I want to caution against reading in to much into these conclusions. The primary target of critique here is not the actions of support worker but the more general structure that designates people with intellectual disabilities as both worthy and incapable of citizenship, as both others and included. Hence, the point is not that we should point fingers towards my interviewees (although it certainly is justified in a few of the examples), but that we must get our heads around how post-institutional politics constitute intellectual disability by a contradiction.

Controlled subjects

The historical, classificatory, and philosophical rationalities of constructing intellectual disability as the otherness of reason means that the LSS, along with other policies of similar ideological origins, produces a situation in which the *outside* of citizenship is figured *within*. As I have shown, the implementation of post-institutional policies of citizenship inclusion responds to this by both relying on governing through citizenship and excluding from citizenship. This corresponds to what we witnessed in the previous two chapters; the inclusion of Taylor and Nussbaum and of the global policy discourse are only possible by re-inscribing exclusion at the instances in which the lack that is attributed to people with intellectual disabilities conflicts with perceptions of citizenship.

Now, this means that we have arrived at a point at which it is possible to formulate how power has transformed after deinstitutionalisation. Together, the technologies of *making* and *restricting* intellectually disabled citizen-subjects create an organisation of disability services that works by control. I argue that this system can be characterised by specifying four prominent features:

1   First, this is a system that *monitors* behaviour. This is a result of the latent need to make decisions concerning if and how to motivate or steer choice making in order for the targeted individuals to comply with the ideals of citizenship. As has been argued by Gilbert (2003), consequential reasoning is a vital characteristic of how individuals monitor their own behaviour. When people with intellectual disabilities are seen as deficient with respect to this capacity, as the interviewees suggest, support workers overtake this monitoring role. Consequently, when people with intellectual disabilities are doing whatever they want, they are *allowed* to do so by someone in a position of authority; if tenants for example are leaving their homes to have a beer, this will generally be preceded by support workers consulting workplace routines, deciding on whether the individual in question can manage to leave the house, deliberating on whether they should be allowed to drink alcohol, pondering the potential consequences, weighing the results of these deliberations against the ethos of the LSS, and thereafter making a decision on how to respond – by standing back, motivating, or using coercive force.

2   This means that the logic of control rests on a *hierarchy* between support workers and tenants: prior to any decision on whether a person with intellectual disability is allowed to have a beer is the positioning of support workers as capable of interfering. The practices of motivation and nurturing citizenship as well as technologies more blatantly departing from the ideals of citizenship are premised on staff having the authority to know what citizenship requires and how a citizen-subject can be accomplished.

3   The regime of control must be *constant* since decisions on technologies of motivation or steering are context and person specific. There is no way of knowing beforehand when a situation that calls for motivation or coercion will arise. This marks an important difference as compared to institutional

care. Strict rules, locked gates, pre-decided menus, and so on were the exemplary technologies of government of the institution. In supported living, these have transformed into practices of micromanagement of individuals. Decisions on courses of action in supported living often regard mundane situations that occur more or less every day: every time a tenant decides on what to eat, to have a cup of coffee, or whether to leave the home, group home staffers are potentially faced with situations that they may believe require steering or motivation. In contrast, when food was cooked and eaten collectively, coffee served at specific times, and leaving the institution forbidden, there was no need for constant monitoring, as appropriate behaviour was largely enforced by collective regulations and restrictions of behaviour.

4   This also implies that control is *individualised*. Since the capacities of citizenship and the likelihood to make what is seen as 'harmful choices' are not seen as evenly distributed within the population of individuals with intellectual disability, control must be adjusted for each person. Thus, we do not see general rules in the group home prohibiting buying one's own clothes. Instead, we see how every employee at each group home is 'responsible' for a tenant, helping them with practical matters provided their understanding of the needs of that particular individual. This requires the creation of personal bonds and detailed knowledge about each individual living in a group home. Sometimes the tenant will be prevented from buying certain clothes, sometimes personnel seek to convince tenants that certain clothes should be bought, and sometimes it means not interfering with which clothes people with intellectual disabilities buy. Therefore, the views and character of the individual support worker will impact how situations are handled. Some might be very likely to intervene, some less.

These are the general features of the decentralised government of post-institutionalisation. In institutional care, the life of the individual was *enclosed* by power and government; it was restricted by rules, constrained by the walls of the institution building, and temporally divided by collectively enforced schedules. In the new regime of simultaneous inclusion and exclusion, the life of the individual is instead *penetrated* by government. The cultivation of citizenship capacities, the enforcement of occasional restrictions, and the application of technologies of motivation require that public officials enter the heads of the individuals that they work with: support workers must be trusted yet seen as authorities; they need to apply individualised technologies to convince, win over, and detract; and they need to be able to estimate when the individuals that they work with can be trusted with self-determination and independence (see Gilbert, 2003).

It is worth noting that only the particular blend of rationales that simultaneously view people with intellectual disabilities as both 'citizens in the making' and 'failed citizens' can produce the microcosm of power described here. During institutionalisation, when individuals with intellectual disability were categorically seen as non-citizens, there was no need for monitoring or deciding on interventions on an individual and constant basis. On the other hand, in a system in which the ideals of citizenship are compatible with the targeted group, this kind of control would not be necessary, since there would be no otherness calling for surveillance in the first place. Instead, such a regime would rely on conformity to social norms (see Foucault, 1990:144). It is only when people with intellectual disabilities are regarded both as potential citizens and as failing to be citizens that the regime of control is activated.

Government of citizenship

A common assumption of much disability research is that citizenship and power are opposites, which means that politics of inclusion serves the purpose of freeing individuals with intellectual disability from power. I believe to have countered this view by showing two things: first, in support work, power flows through relations between staff and individuals with intellectual disability in the form of 'motivation' and nurturing of capacities, along the lines of the support worker's ideas of what citizenship entails. Thus, although seeing their support work as congruent with the politics of citizenship inclusion, this clearly cannot be seen as the absence of power. Second, coercion and restrictions, when occurring, are not remnants of the past but correspond to the idea that people with this diagnosis lack capacities necessary for self-determination and independence. In supported living, making decisions for people of this group recurs and is integrated into the service provision of most group homes that I have visited. It is hence a vital aspect which is entrenched in how supported living functions. Thus, directly countering the ambitions of government withdrawal from the lives of people with intellectual disabilities, post-institutionalisation meant an intensification of government, constant, individualised, and penetrative in how public officials attempt to enter the mind of the individual.

Deleuze (1992:3–5) has argued that towards the end of the 20th century, 'control' was on the verge of becoming a new paradigmatic mode of government, succeeding disciplinary institutions and replacing them with calculus and surveillance of flows of individuals. Not considering the wider implications and merits of this argument, he stresses that a disciplinary regime means that the individual ceaselessly starts again, 'from school to the barracks, from the barracks, to the factory' (Deleuze, 1992:3), and so on. In contrast, in a society of control 'one is never finished' (5). This certainly seems to say something of importance concerning the control of people with intellectual disabilities, who are always monitored, being worked on, nurtured, in order to become what they are not. The processes of never-ending nurturing and restricting are instigated by the predicament of post-institutionalisation: whilst institutionalisation was designed to separate and discipline the otherness of human reason, politics of inclusion works by moulding such others into citizens and to simultaneously retract their rights in situations in which they are seen as incapable. It will never be finished, since the very constitution of intellectual disability means that people of this group are defined by lacking capacities of citizenship.

Remember here that a basic theoretical proposition of this book is that citizenship requires a certain kind of subject: the subject of humanism that went into the constitution of intellectual disability when this group first emerged. But as intellectual disability remains outside this notion of what characterises human beings, efforts of inclusion will be ridden with conflicts and tension, disruptions and supplements that end up in a politics of simultaneous inclusion and exclusion. In this way, the biopolitics of the post-institutional era is both founded on and haunted by the instability of the structure of inclusion/exclusion; it needs designations of otherness in order to direct interventions, but it also needs government by inclusion to craft a self-ruling citizenry. Hence, if the first and introductory part of the book established how intellectual disability consolidated the otherness of humanist reason as a diagnosis, attached with certain pre-political characteristics, the chapters of this part have examined how a regime of citizenship making continuously seeks and fails to incorporate such naturalised otherness. It follows that the politics of post-institutionalisation cannot be made sense of in the terminologies that presently dominate disability politics, of 'emancipation' as 'citizenship', of 'power' as the opposite of 'freedom', and of 'inclusion'/'exclusion' as a dichotomous and mutually excluding pair. The way that people with this condition are being governed does not fit with our inherited theoretical vocabularies.

To summarise the movement that I have described throughout the book and up to this point, the emergence of 'intellectual disability' was a response to how some people did not fit into the separation of the humanist subject from non-human living things. Before classification and modern medicine, these people were part of an unnamed melange of various groups that were seen as occupying the space between humans and animals. Consider, for example, how Clifford Simplican (2015) discusses the insecure positioning of 'idiots' and 'changelings' in Locke's philosophy, neither fully human nor beasts. Biopolitics attempted to govern this constitutive outside: classification would name them 'mentally deficient' and similar and designate them as 'others' of human reason. They were incorporated into binary schemes of inclusion/exclusion, normal/pathological, and reason/lack of reason. Thus, the unruly constitutive outside was tamed and managed, confined and removed from the rest of society as targets of the politics of exclusion. When government set out to once again include this group, however, without reconsidering its constitution as the defining outside of the ideals of citizenship, it gives rise to a politics in which this group is simultaneously being both inside and outside of the sphere of citizenship. Hence, people with intellectual disabilities again appear as an extreme that eludes the prevailing conception of politics, this time neither 'excluded' nor 'included' but both.

Notes

1 The past two or three years have seen some worrying tendencies linked to politics of austerity. At the time of finishing this book, the costs of disability services were being debated, and a public commission had been appointed to evaluate the functioning of the LSS and of personal assistance in particular. The disability movement is very critical and worried about these developments.
2 When the LSS was introduced, personal assistance was the service getting most popular attention, not least because it was strongly advocated by the disability movement and

emerged from the ideology of 'independent living'. The reason why it is not studied here is that supported living is far more common for people with intellectual disabilities.

3 Other studies, notably Clement and Bigby's (2010), have other models for differentiating between forms of supported living, for example separating group homes from individual apartments where individuals are not renting their apartments from the same organisation that provides services. The reason why such distinctions are not made here is that the Swedish system has both pure group homes (although the persons living in them are 'tenants', legally speaking), 'stairwell living units' without shared areas, and satellite apartments tied to nearby personal units. Oftentimes, staffers are working with tenants living in a group home, as well as with the tenants of a few satellite appartments, which renders it difficult to distinguish between these different service forms in the interviews.

4 For a similar example from the Netherlands, see Schipper et al. (2011:529–30).

5 See Yates et al. (2008:254) for similar descriptions of restrictions of the freedom of movement.

Part III
Resistance

6 Vulnerability

The theorisation of the biopolitics of intellectual disability, of post-institutionalisation, urges us to ask: What next? How can we theorise beyond the imposed limitations of this regime of power? How can it be resisted against? There are two main purposes of the following three chapters. The first one is to describe how present intellectual disability politics is contested. In this respect, it will be impossible for me to come even remotely close to a complete picture. Rather, I aim to examine some instances of resistance that allow me to pinpoint theoretical ideas concerning how the present regime of government can be rethought. Thus, second, I want to draw on the instances of resistance examined in order to arrive at a set of critical analytical tools that can serve as resources in challenges of the politics of post-institutionalisation. In this chapter, I will examine how support workers resist citizenship inclusion by mobilising an identity as 'carers', the next chapter discusses how political activists diagnosed with intellectual disability engage in representational politics, and, last, Chapter 8 presents an analysis of how a discourse of 'ethics' frames attempts to contest present policies of prenatal diagnosis.

As we shall see, the instances of resistance that are focused in these three chapters emerge as inclusion and exclusion come into friction. Thus, the mobilisation of 'caring work', opposed to citizenship politics, arises as support workers recognise a gap between promises of inclusion and a perceived lack in the people that they work with; the representational politics of intellectual disability transpires as activists demand that their ascription of citizenship status should also entitle them to political self-organisation; and contestations of prenatal diagnosis must be understood against the background of the rift between common ascriptions of equal human value and screening practices which effectuate the prevention of intellectual disability. The reason why spaces of resistance open up at precisely these points is that the prevailing discourse does not seem to add up; it presents itself as sanctimonious, which means that processes of questioning, challenging, and reassessing can take off. This is the first part of the argument: that the simultaneity of inclusion/exclusion described in previous chapters creates spaces for contestation. The second part is that resistance against the biopolitical regime comes with both promises of progress and threats of consolidation of the regime of power. Hence, we shall for example see how the discourse of 'care' is integrated into the present governmental system as a justification of paternalism, but, at the same time, the notion of 'care' may also lead us to consider vulnerability as a constitutive feature of human being, thereby destabilising the dichotomous division between 'able' and 'disabled'. Similarly, politics of representation carries both the promise of self-representation and the threat of essentialism, and the 'ethical' framing of debates about prenatal diagnosis both works to de-politicise this practice and can point towards the re-politicisation of ethics itself.

However, to get these arguments going, I first need to devote a few odd pages to set the stage by introducing some theoretical starting points surrounding the elusive notions of 'resistance' and 'critique'.

Power and resistance

Throughout, 'biopolitics' has been my primary theoretical term when discussing the government of intellectual disability. It is therefore apt to focus my discussion of resistance on Foucault. It follows from the general theoretical starting points of this book that 'resistance', just as power, is a complex and dispersed phenomenon. This can be illustrated by Foucault's (1980:142) interpretation of their relationship:

> there are no relations of power without resistances; the latter are all the more real and effective because they are formed right at the point where relations of power are exercised; resistance to power does not have to come from elsewhere to be real, nor is it inexorably frustrated through being the compatriot of power.

As indicated here, power and resistance cannot be understood as dichotomous forces, clashing in struggles over the future. Rather, the reason why resistance appears everywhere we find power is that power itself is never completely free-floating and devoid of friction with the societies and subjects it shapes. Thus, resistance and power are coexistent: power will always encounter resistance, and resistance requires a force to resist. In Foucault's thinking, power and resistance are ontologically similar: like power, resistance emerges from everywhere, which means that dominating social movements, radical political parties, and the like are not the only places, perhaps not even the most important ones, where contestations emerge. Furthermore, and as we shall see in the discussions that will follow, since resistance emerges in tandem with systems of government and within its discursive and structural confines, it easily ends up reproducing what it aims to overthrow.

During the latter years of his life, Foucault developed these ideas into comprehension of resistance as a way of governing oneself. Whereas he previously, and quite straightforwardly, had denoted subjects as effects of discourse and power, he came to refine his analysis to describe that subjects come into being *in relation to* discourses, norms, and institutions, thus implying room for agency (see Foucault, 2010:41–74; 2011:23–32). We cannot act unaffected by power, but this does not imply that we are determined and that our actions are the result of causal forces. Essentially, this points towards the possibility of navigating fields of action in order to come into being beyond the confines of the rationalities of government (see Hartmann, 2003). Foucault's (1997:101–34) follow-up on Kant's (1991[1784]) 'An Answer to the Question: "What is Enlightenment?"' is especially interesting in this context. In his identically entitled paper, he identifies in Kant's analysis of human limitations of knowledge the seeds for a critical attitude which can simultaneously examine and transgress the boundaries of what is possible to think. Kant's notion of 'critique' thus transforms into a call to examine the history of the forces that have shaped the limits of our thinking, an exercise that may open up the possibility of transcending these limits. In other words, resistance is intimately linked to the notion of critique, which in this context means interrogating the limits that systems of power impose on our thinking and doing. From this perspective, there will always be spaces where thinking and doing differently is possible; cracks in systems of rule that can be activated and used as springboards for alternative ways of existing (see Simons, 1995:90). As Butler (2005:17) has formulated it, the shaping of subjectivity can also be a site of critique.

Hence, as Simons (1995:81) notes, subjects are always enmeshed by relations of power but never completely subsumed, always limited but never trapped. Critique as a form of resistance transforms the limiting nature of power to become a starting point for re-examining who we are (see Simons, 1995:17); in other words, by understanding contestations of post-institutional intellectual disability politics, we may find ways of thinking that unsettle prevailing ideas about this group and how its members should be treated.

Caring resistance

As previously shown, contemporary intellectual disability politics simultaneously constitutes and restricts citizen subjects. In the remainder of this chapter, I will analyse how support workers depart from the ethos of citizenship, frequently described by the interviewees in the previous chapter, as a form of decentralised resistance against the formal goals of politics of inclusion. When support workers suspend the law they are also contesting it, delineating its reach, and countering its explicit purposes. As I will argue, the recurring circumventions of the legislation are motivated by a uniform set of values and beliefs, expressed by support workers as being involved in emotional, almost family-like relationships with tenants. Hence, in contrast to the formally sanctioned relationship between a citizen and a public servant, support workers activate another discourse that enables another set of actions in order to sidestep formal regulations. It is a form of resistance that arises as a reaction against the nurturing of intellectually disabled individuals to become self-regulating citizens, it is decentralised in how it is not tied to any specific movement, organisation, or coordinated plan, and it is best analysed as a set of interrelated discursive and enacted constructions.

Examining this, I will argue two things. *First*, legitimising coercion and challenging liberal citizenship by reference to one's informal and emotionally entangled relationship to tenants reinforces the belief that people with intellectual disabilities are distinctively 'other' in relation to an all-embracing imagined 'normality' bound up with rights of self-determination and autonomy. Thus, this form of resistance serves to reinforce the overarching biopolitical logic of simultaneous inclusion and exclusion. *Second*, however, the interviews also highlight a boundary of liberal thinking that is important by merit of what may lie beyond it. The narratives of emotional engagement direct attention to a dimension of caring, as practice and attitude, which needs to be explored for its potential to unsettle presumed assumptions concerning the humanist subject and disability politics. I shall conclude the chapter by discussing this limit in light of recent developments in feminist and disability theory coalescing around the notion of 'vulnerability', arguing that intellectual disability is an expression of how human beings are 'doubly vulnerable'.

Justifying coercion

The analysis that follows builds on the same material as the previous chapter, here focusing specifically on how support workers justify their departures from the legislation and the ideals of citizenship. To start with, the group home is a place of *public* work carried out in the *home*, helping individuals to sort out their hygiene, make food, and take their medications. This means that the border between private and public, so central to traditional understandings of state responsibility in liberal democracies, is considerably blurred from the outset. This border is not only traversed as concerns *what* staffers do and *where* they do it but also concerning *how* they see their own role and principal task.

> In this job, it is much like a home. They are people, you know. We are with them in their everyday lives so of course I take with me my personal beliefs and views upon life.
>
> (AP10)

> I think that people [with intellectual disability] are developing [from close relations with personnel]. We are their arms – we are their family. Unfortunately, that's how it is. We work intensively with them all the time. They probably know more about us than our own parents. Some of them have followed staff home to celebrate Christmas – we don't get paid for it, but we want to do it.
>
> (AP8)

These quotes showcase a way of looking at work that seems alien to traditional notions of the civil servant. Importantly, in the material, the traversed border between a professional role and an informal one recurs when the interviewees try to legitimise actions that break with the formal regulations. At these instances, the interviewees no longer talk of themselves as public servants but as having formed emotional bonds with tenants that they are acting on. In this way, throughout the material, when the support workers are to justify actions that break with the LSS and the ethos of citizenship inclusion, they enter the role of the emotionally motivated protector; this role operates as a means of resistance against citizenship politics.

As I will discuss at some length in this chapter, the interviewees often appeal to an ethics which echoes feminist notions of care, as developed by Carol Gilligan (1982), Joan Tronto (1993), Selma Sevenhuijsen (1998, 2003), and others. This literature contests the instrumental reasoning of liberal philosophy by emphasising 'caring' as a specific class of actions and attitudes transmitting a specific ethos and its target of criticism is the narrowness of view in mainstream moral and political philosophy (Pettersen, 2011:61). In the interviews, it often appears that switching from a formal role as a public servant to an emotionally invested informal role as a 'carer' is motivated by a deeply felt cognitive dissonance on behalf of the support workers:

> There is a responsibility to follow the law, but also a responsibility to cater to their well being. It becomes so frustrating . . . But I feel that if they live here, they are not fully capable. In that case, they also have a right to be cared for, to get the best care there is.
>
> (BP2)

In this way, watching the people one works with make 'bad' decisions causes distress and bad conscience. In such situations, support workers tend to empathise with the ascribed suffering of the people they work with. However, acting on this paternalistic impulse is not possible as long as their formal role of implementing the law is understood as the primary source of legitimation. As seen in the previous quote, 'caring' is juxtaposed with the self-determination and independence associated with the law; it offers different grounds for legitimation.

The shift to a caring role is marked by a number of recurring characteristics. When acting against the self-determination of people with intellectual disabilities, the interviewees see themselves as (1) *emotionally* tied to the people they work with, (2) personally *responsible* for their safety and as acting based on an (3) *informal* rather than a formal relationship. In addition, (4) they come to focus on the *individual* and their suffering rather than on overarching principles of justice, and they do so based on the presumption that they have (5) *superior knowledge* as to which choices are wise and which are not. In sum, this means that meetings between staffers and people who have been granted the right to supported living are no longer seen as involving 'public servants' and 'citizens' but rather as following the structure of parental relationships.

Now, since feelings of attachment and responsibility are hard to fit into a conceptual framework founded on individualism and procedural justice, the depictions of an emotionally ridden relationship with tenants point towards what is perceived as a limit of citizenship. Whilst citizenship implies rule of law and formal rights, in extension leading to an impartial and rule-bound rationality where there is a firm line of demarcation separating individual freedom and state power, here, the justifications of constraint rather expose a logic of action organised around commitment, empathy, and protection. In the interviews, this is repeatedly described by the metaphor of a 'family':

> How do you handle such situations with your kids, what they are allowed to eat and what are they allowed to do and not do? I am not allowing my kids to go out in shorts in the middle of the winter. I cannot allow the people I work with here do that either, just because they are supposed to be 'self-determined' and 'independent'.
>
> (AP8)

> Well, self-determination . . . surely, we do that as long as it works. But we eat together here, for example, so they do not get to choose what to eat every day. No one here can have food in his or her own refrigerator, because it will be gone the next morning. And the people living here enjoy eating together, although there might be some bickering around the table, it is more like a family. The staff are sitting together and eating with them, although we have brought our own food, so we all eat together. Sometimes they ask us what we are eating and if they can have a bite, and of course they can. We have worked with them for such a long time that we really know them well.
>
> (AP4)

The 'family' metaphor operates by incorporating the norm system of the family, for example in disallowing one's kids to eat whatever they like, into the context of publicly regulated disability services. In the first quote, the interviewee seemingly understands that the LSS does not authorise her deciding whether to allow tenants to wear shorts or not. However, as a mother, this kind of coercion is perfectly appropriate. In order for this particular support worker to be able to legitimately make decisions over this person labelled with intellectual disability, she transforms her self-identity into that of a 'parent', which in turn legitimises her paternalistic decision making.[1]

In summary: the circumventions of citizenship rights that restrict people with intellectual disabilities are very rarely expressions of malice or indifference but are, to the contrary, framed as expressions of commitment and concern stemming from emotional engagement. It is resistance against citizenship politics, where support workers counter its purposes and ideals. By extension, an ethics of care supplements the disruption that emerges when intellectual disability meets the ideal of citizenship inclusion. Repeatedly in the interviews, the ideals of citizenship are depicted as removed from practical day-to-day matters, as stale and overly rigorous in relation to work in supported living. The same way that the ethics of care challenges a moral ontology of self-sufficient individuals striving to be independent, the interviewees draw on a similar set of values to contest these ideas as expressed in disability legislation. As the interviews reveal, the language of rights and professionalism is seen as unable to account for the multitude of feelings, anxieties, and conflicting intuitions that emerge in group home work.

The ideology of citizenship in present disability politics depicts the state apparatus as a constant threat of individual freedom. This is why rights are needed as safeguards against state infringements, why the state must be restrained in order to be legitimate, and hence also why this tradition is not very well prepared to handle the kind of relationships that are described by the support workers. It is against this ideological background that the stories of the support workers must be understood. Their resistance is located at the limits of liberal conceptions of citizenship, depicting a kind of relationship that has no evident place in the dominating story of how citizens and the state are related.

Reinforcing biopolitics

Although the support workers surely are exercising resistance, this is not resistance against the broader biopolitical regime of government. Rather, what we see here is a form of resistance that ultimately works to effectuate the overarching logic of the present government of intellectual disability. As Foucault (1990) contends, government is not a straightforward, top-down, or unilateral activity. Rather, government is made up of numerous different actors, with different agendas, that are generating different kinds of power/resistance relationships (see Rose, 1999:19). This is why the resistance of the support workers can both deter the flows of power of the politics of citizenship *and* reinforce the more general biopolitical logic of concurrent inclusion and exclusion.

Consider here the working conditions of street-level support workers. The fact that they can shortcut the legislation without authorisation testifies to a substantial amount of room for discretionary decision making (see Lipsky, 1980). This can be interpreted as a result of lack of detailed regulations, control, and sanctions when the law is superseded. It can be interpreted as *absence*. There are no institutionalised and systematic controlling mechanisms, for example, and very few evaluation tools to measure the extent to which the goals of the law are met in everyday support work. The absence of direct steering and control, however, does not testify to the *absence* of government. To the contrary, the lack of steering has its own governmental logic of allowing discretion; the *absence* of regulation and the allowance of discretion constitutes a form of government which operates by *neglecting* to intervene in the instances where the promise of citizenship is withdrawn. The fact that there seems to be a general awareness that the law is not being followed and that the legislation is circumvented exposes this logic: it is a mode of government which allows the promise of citizenship to be broken, effectuating all of the small interventions into the individual autonomy of people with intellectual disabilities. These are neither mistakes nor examples of deliberate evil but a structural feature of the government of disability. It is a form of steering which relies on the absence of formal steering and thus allows for the disruption of intellectual disability to be handled at the lowest level of policy implementation.

Accordingly, the ambiguous positioning of people with intellectual disabilities as being both entitled to citizenship and the defining others of citizenship is ultimately handled where a leeway to cope with the contradictory status of the group exists. If giving and retracting 'citizenship' characterise post-institutionalisation, the emotional engagement expressed by the interviewees serves to justify the retraction. The space for support workers to resist, emerging in the rift between the rights and defining lack of people with intellectual disabilities, is thus ultimately used in ways that revert to a notion of this condition as marked by inferiority. In the stories of the interviews, recognising the dependency of others never amounts to recognising dependency and vulnerability in oneself. This begs the question: if 'caring resistance' works to uphold the biopolitics of intellectual disability, might there still be something of value to it that can point beyond this regime of government?

Vulnerable subjects

If the first argument of this chapter concerned paternalism as resistance against citizenship, the second argument – that I will elaborate on in what follows – engages the presumed dichotomy between 'independence' and 'dependence' and the notion of 'vulnerability' in order to explore the opportunities of mobilising critique and resistance beyond the confines of the present biopolitical regime. In other words, how can we theorise at the limit of liberal citizenship – the very limit that the interviews directed us to – without reverting to re-inscribe a constitutive and pre-political lack of people with intellectual disabilities?

Independence and vulnerability

As was hinted at above, the ethics of care attempts to highlight an ignored dimension of mainstream political discourse concerning human relationships, namely that 'care' is never a one-directional activity involving a caregiver and someone dependent on the care but an activity binding people together through our interdependencies. As Hettema (2014) points out, the ethics of care seeks to set up a framework for thinking about justice that opposes and highlights the limitations of the individualism which permeates present Western societies – the same limits, I argue, that the interviewees seek to push by mobilising an identity as informal caregivers. Central to this philosophical project is a relational ontology that sees humans as dependent on care in order to be caring toward others (Fine, 2004:218; Pettersen, 2011:55, 58). This insight has led care ethicists to reflect on human relationships in terms that come close to the emotional commitment exposed in the interviews, highlighting context, dependency, and engagement. However, opposed to how the interviewees justify their paternalism, the theoretical work on care seeks to depart from a binary division between 'carers' and 'care receivers', instead arguing that everyone, in principle, is capable of providing care and that everyone at some point will receive care (Sevenhuijsen, 2003:184).

A central point of the ethics of care is its critique of the presumed oppositional relationship between 'independence' and 'dependence'. Instead of seeing these as strict opposites, dependency on caring relations is analysed as a precondition of independence. In taking this view, acting on the vulnerability of others means that we are simultaneously providing their basis to function as autonomous and purposeful individuals. Thereby, the firm separation between those in need of help and those who are living 'independently' is undone. This conflicts with how independence/dependence is understood within the overarching norm sources of the politics of post-institutionalisation, where 'dependency' is often presumed to represent powerlessness, exposure, and a lack of control (see Verstraete, 2007; WHO, 2011:37, 263). This often taken-for-granted ideological starting point has important implications for how we understand certain critiques of ethics of care directed from within disability studies and, more importantly, as concerns the place of 'independence'/'dependence' in debates about disability politics more generally. The accusation that caring ethics ascribes 'dependency' relies on the presumption that 'independence' is superior and the norm. When a prominent disability scholar such as Oliver (1996:65) declares that 'dependency' is an effect of discriminating social, economic, and political forces, he takes the liberal yardstick of 'independence' for granted, failing to acknowledge a more fundamental kind of dependency which is integral to the human condition. This is a mode of critique that fails to address the ontological underpinnings of what it criticises. The proposal that humans are intrinsically dependent as interdependent beings challenges not only the liberal ideals inherent to disability legislations but also the ideological underpinnings of much research on disability that attempts to critically assess these legislations. To be able to develop this into a positive notion of human relationships, however, we also need to account for how some disability scholars have theorised human vulnerability.

Within disability studies, and from theoretical positions similar to my own, some scholars have sought to draw on 'vulnerability' to destabilise the firm separation between 'interdependent' and 'dependent', 'able' and 'disabled', stressing that we all go through phases of dependence in our lives, whether we are labelled 'disabled' or not (see Davis, 2002:3; Scully, 2014:218). For individuals under stood as 'normal', our universal dependency most often goes unacknowledged. After all, most people in Western societies are dependent on things such as the availability of food in our local stores, on our phones operating as expected, on public transportation running smoothly, on public information targeting us in times of crisis, and on dental care to take care of our teeth when they hurt. Every one of these examples presupposes a functioning supply chain, where numerous others are necessary in order for us to uphold a 'normal' way of life (see Scully, 2014:215). Yet none of these examples are acknowledged as 'dependence' in a politically relevant sense. As a political term, 'dependence' has come to denote ways of living and being that are associated with individuals who are separated from what is considered 'normal' (see Fraser & Gordon, 1997). This is why 'dependence' on functioning public transportation is only acknowledged as such when it concerns disabled peoples' access of riding the bus using wheelchairs, whilst it goes unacknowledged for 'normal' people commuting to work. The line of division here is made up of the prior judgement that people with disability are a special category of human being, a certain class requiring special attention, whose needs and views are repeatedly ignored when things such as public transportation are in the planning stages.

When we start to see our own lives, or any life, in light of the fluctuating needs we all have, we are provided with the opportunity to question the distribution of independence/dependence, how certain dependencies are understood as 'bad' and how these serve as the constitutive outside of the valued position of 'independence'. Thus, Kittay's argument that 'dependency' is 'grounded in the inevitable circumstances of the human animal' (Kittay, 2003:260) directs attention towards how we all fall short of ideals of full ability and complete independence. Provided this insight, disability can be understood as a consequence of our biology being fragile and open to injury when encountering the world (see Siebers, 2008:7), in turn suggesting that 'disability gathers us into the everyday community of embodied humankind' (Garland Thomson, 2012). Basically, disability is a reminder of what it means to have a body that exists in a world of things that appear to be external to it, which is to suggest that the vulnerabilities and dependencies associated with disability cannot be separated from 'normal living' (see Siebers, 2008:5; Scully, 2014). Garland Thomson (2012) has pointed out that the script of fully normal development is a path very few of us can follow for an extended period of time. Most of us are, in some stage of life, temporarily disabled. The construction of 'disability' as a designation of a specific group thus obscures how disability is a shared experience, constantly making inroads into 'normality', and a lurking possibility and potentiality in all of us. Not un-poetically, Garland Thomson (2012:342) formulates this latent potentiality as bearing 'witness to our inherent receptiveness, to being shaped by the particular journey through the world that we call our life'.

In this way, disability is not alien to normality but an integral part of what it means to be human. At the same time, it is also firmly separated in order to protect the ideals of full functionality and independence. In this context, Garland Thomson (2006:262) writes of a societal 'will to normalize', to rid life of all unpredictability and non-conformity by means of regulation and control of deviancy. For Susan Wendell (2006:247–9) this stems from our unwillingness and our incapacity to confront our own bodies, which we cannot accept as fragile and open to injury (see Davis, 2002:3–4). Hence, our cultural insistence to control the body shifts blame onto people with disability for failing at this task, and so this particular form of otherness comes to embody our universal failure to meet the ideals of 'independence' and ability. By these processes, our universal vulnerabilities are hidden by being projected onto groups that stand as examples of what 'dependency' is and looks like. In this masquerade, the intellectually disabled subject appears as the removed expressions of our lack of reason, faltering cognition, emerging dementia, and so on, removing these traits from the sphere of normalcy. Kristeva (2010:251) calls this 'a *narcissistic identity wound* in the person who is not disabled' and goes on to state of the non-disabled person that 'he inflicts a threat of *physical or physical death*, fear of collapse, and, beyond that, the anxiety of seeing the very *borders of the human species* explode'. In a less theoretically dense formulation, Goodley (2014:38) states that 'disability reminds ability of its own vulnerability', appearing as a threat– indeed, a psychological one at that, I would add, to our ontological foundations. Hence, when the norm of the reasonable brain, the self-sufficient master of one's own life, is constructed and contrasted to the otherness of intellectual disability, the threat is simultaneously handled and created, producing both the assurance the dependency associated with a lack of reason is somewhere else and the possibility that the difference between 'us' and 'them' is not as firm as it seems. This is akin to what Butler (1993:26–7) calls 'the spectre of a terrifying return', in this context describing how disability haunts normality by threatening its coherence and reasonableness. The sustained efforts to remove intellectual disability and to distinguish it as a qualitatively different class of human existence is a way of keeping the terrifying return at bay.

Doubly vulnerable

Now, I believe that this line of reasoning can ultimately provoke us to reconsider the phenomenon of intellectual disability as such – indeed, that it can help us move beyond the clash of nature and politics that I discussed at the end of Chapter 2 as the ever-present theoretical framing in debates revolving around the ontology of disability.

The vulnerability stressed by Garland Thomson, Goodley, Davis, and Wendell emerges in the interface between body and world. I believe that this only tells half of the story: although these disability theorists successfully highlight the potential of 'vulnerability' in order to deconstruct the division between 'able' and 'disabled', their accounts downplay an equally important aspect of what the notion of vulnerability can lead us to suggest, namely that it also concerns how our bodily constitutions are always made sense of in discourse and that we emerge as subjects through social categorisations. The cultural nexus of ideas about disability, denoting it as a special category and difference of sorts, and the assemblage of governmental technologies developed to handle these differences all represent aspects of the social and political entanglement with biology that I analysed with respect to classification, psychiatry, and medicine. And it is precisely by means of such social frames of interpretation, constructed in language, that we are able to understand the bodily fragilities that constitute us as vulnerable beings.

As I believe that this is somewhat new theoretical ground, expanding on already rather complex arguments, I shall try to tread carefully. In *Excitable Speech*, Butler (1997:1–2) examines the implications of understanding subjectivity as constructed in language, stating that such constitution exposes a fundamental vulnerability stemming from the fact that discourse conditions our being. In Althusser's (1971 in Butler, 1997:24) wording, the speech act inaugurating the subject precedes the subject (see Butler, 1997:24). This suggests that the terminologies through which we know ourselves and our relations to others are never of our own making. Indeed, as Butler (1997:26) develops, there can be no protection against a call into existence that appears in language and which is necessary in order to consolidate our identities. Therefore, we may cling to the terminology that constructs who we are and designates our social existence (Butler, 1997:26). In essence, this implies that subjects are always constituted in discourses beyond their own control. In the context of this chapter, this is to suggest that the categories of 'able' and 'disabled' necessarily precondition how we make sense of human vulnerabilities, how we neglect and hide them by projecting them onto certain people categorised along the lines of 'normal' and 'deviant'. In other words, the fundamental human vulnerability which stems from our bodily encounters with the world will be intertwined with an equally fundamental vulnerability that stems from these encounters always being made sense of in discourses that precedes our emergence as subjects (see Butler, 1997:4; 2004:43).

Now, Butler (2005:35–6) talks of this as 'exposure' with respect to discourse in order to highlight how other people, equally exposed, are always implied in these processes of subject formation. As the categories that people with intellectual disabilities come to inhabit are naturalised, there is little chance of escaping the associated terminology of 'disorder', 'cognitive deficit', and 'risk'. At the same time, this very language and its underlying normativity provide the justification of seeking to erase intellectual disability by prenatal diagnosis, new drugs, or genetic counselling showing how this is ultimately a question of existence and extinction (see, Taylor, 2013). To exemplify this, consider here how the authority of norms, institutions, sciences, laws, and regulations are all brought to bear on subjectivities being shaped. Consider how these apparatuses construct intellectual disability, how people with this condition are medically defined and diagnosed through the language of 'intelligence' and adaptive behaviour tests; how routines and local regulations pin down which behaviours are considered to be acceptable in a group home and how they are related to a set of associations, ideas, and propositions of the condition. As Hettema (2014:495) points out, such frameworks precede our actions, are of a higher order than our preferences, and therefore appear to be external to us; it is a network of discourses through which being becomes possible, at times impossible, and even when we pass as 'normal', the very division between 'them and 'us' will condition our being.

Thus, we are dealing with two aspects of vulnerability: on the one hand, stemming from the fragility of when body meets world and, on the other, from our fundamental exposure towards the discursive preconditions of subjectivity. Now, I suggest that 'intellectual disability' emerges at the point where bodily and discursive vulnerability become inseparable: it is both the friction of brain meeting world and the sense making of this process by means of discourse. This interlinking can be elucidated by again utilising the proposition that every statement of a body functions as a further formation of that body (Butler, 1993: xix): the very act of describing a bodily vulnerability as a 'disability' contributes to constituting that body as 'disabled', which represents the discursive vulnerability. Thus, people with disabilities are vulnerable, as we all are, not only by their bodies interacting with the world in unexpected ways but also this interaction is made comprehensible through a set of ideas that constitute them as 'deviant', 'other', and fundamentally different. And in this way, people with intellectual disabilities can be understood as 'doubly vulnerable', not because they are especially vulnerable but because they expose how subjects come into being provided the intertwinement of our exposure towards the world and towards how we make sense of this provided the power of knowledge and discourse.

To conclude this argument, I argued earlier that disability could be seen as a projection of the universal failure to meet ideals of independence and full functionality onto a specific group. This, of course, also holds for people with intellectual disabilities, whose brains meet the world and its social organisation in ways that have resulted in their removal from the sphere of 'normalcy'. However, I also think that intellectual disability can be made sense of as a result of a parallel removal of our discursive vulnerability. Thus, the same way that our bodily exposure is handled by removal, there is a similar removal with respect to our vulnerability as constituted through language. The implication of Butler's analysis of how subjects come into being in relation to discourse is that human beings are fundamentally incapable of reaching narrative closure, since they are unable to explain how they became an 'I' capable of telling their own story (see Butler, 2005:37). This rendering of subjectivity clearly contradicts the ideal of the humanist subject, which is transcendental to *him*self (for the humanist subject is gendered) and able to tell his own story, coherently and effortlessly. This means that Butler essentially suggests that we are all fundamentally incomplete with respect to the ideals of humanist reason. In turn, just like our universal incompleteness with respect to ideals of full bodily functionality, discursive vulnerability is handled by removal and projection onto a specific group that come to stand in for our universal failure to meet this ideal. This is 'the intellectually disabled subject', which appears to mask how we are all displaced by language and thus lack full control of our own identity.

To summarise this discussion: the medico-political categories of 'disability', 'intellectual disability', and so forth rest on an untenable separation between independence and dependence. Rather, as several disability theorists have argued, vulnerability is a common trait to humanity, not only specific to those we understand as being 'disabled'. As a consequence, disability is not alien to 'normal' life but represents a latent possibility that will sooner or later become manifest but which simultaneously poses a threat to the ideal that human beings are independent. The very act of dealing with this threat, by removing vulnerability from common humanity and projecting it onto certain subjects constituted as 'disabled' is achieved by discourse and hence represents our vulnerability towards the social conditions and discursive frames within which subjects emerge. Intellectual disability can therefore be understood as an outcome of the overlap of discursive and bodily vulnerabilities.

However, this is not to suggest that we should ignore that this group differs, to say that 'intellectual disability' does not exist or that I seek to collapse their specificity into common humanity. Rather, I have argued that we should approach difference differently: instead of understanding some differences that we label 'disabilities', as tied to a pre-set division between 'independence' and 'dependence', I suggest that we see ourselves in the differences represented by the labels of 'disability' and 'intellectual disability', acknowledging the latent possibility of disability in ourselves. Neither is this to call for an appropriation of disabled identity or an attempt to bridge the difference between 'us' and 'them'. Rather, I want to stress the contingent nature of the separation between 'disability' and 'norm'. Hence, instead of only searching for the proper needs of 'dependents' and the political measures through which their needs can be met, I want to ask that careful attention be directed at the instances, appearing in all of us, when the division between 'independence' and 'dependence' breaks down. Following such a route, I believe, represents a mode of critique and resistance that may be able to do what the 'caring resistance' of support workers fails to: to shake the division between 'them' and 'us'.

Note

1 This is similar to how Clement and Bigby (2010:124) describes 'parent–child interactions' in UK group homes.

7 Representation

The material of this chapter consists of a three-hour conversation with activists representing the board and national secretariat of the Swedish self-advocacy organisation Grunden. Although I had never met the activists participating in this particular conversation before, I had followed their work since I got involved with disability politics, and I was familiar with activists of the organisation's local branch in my hometown. The discussion revolved around the relationship between notions of 'representation' and resistance against the prevailing politics of intellectual disability.[1] Partly, this was a result of me assuming that issues of self-representation were important to members of the first Swedish self-advocacy group of people with intellectual disabilities. However, the discussion also revolved around representation, because the activists brought up and returned to this theme throughout.

Three related aspects of 'representation' were central. First, that 'representation' is about self-advocacy and that Grunden, as an organisation, is led by intellectually disabled individuals who represent themselves, which, of course, actualises the thorny issue of who can speak for people of disenfranchised groups. Second, representation is brought up as an issue of how 'intellectual disability' is depicted and, thus, how activists labelled as such both relate to and resist these representations. In the activists' stories, acts of re-presenting what a diagnosis of intellectual disability implies are central to how they understand themselves as political agents. Last, a repeated occurrence during our conversation was that the activists played with, questioned, and unsettled the supposed dividing line and hierarchy between me, the presumably able-brained researcher, and themselves, in ways that came to alter my relation to my own scholarly and political work. I will elaborate on all of these themes throughout.

As we shall see, in parallel to the previous chapter, there are dangers and possibilities surrounding representation. The politics of being seen, heard, and able to voice one's opinions, offer both the opportunity to transgress and the threat of reifying, cultural presumptions about intellectual disability. Also, like in the previous and the coming chapter, the purpose of engaging these dangers and possibilities is to find ways of theorising intellectual disability in new ways. In this chapter, this is largely a shared task between me and the activists, which means that the text that follows is written and structured differently than the rest of this book, indeed, that the very notion of 'theory' as a resource of sense making becomes something else. Rather than the authoritative 'voice of the researcher', I have sought to engage in a conversation in which the search for conclusions is a shared task, in which ambiguities are allowed to come to the fore, and in which I have abstained from editing or cutting out when the people I talk to are questioning my vantage point.

Monica:	Is it ok if we take some pictures and put them on our Facebook?
Niklas:	Absolutely.
Monica:	We document everything when someone is visiting us.
Niklas:	Perhaps you are getting quite used to being visited?
Monica:	Oh yes, we are.
Andrea:	There are really lots of people interested . . .
Niklas:	I can see that. I wanted to quickly present myself again. As you probably remember from my e-mail and our phone calls, I started to take interest in the politics of intellectual disability when working in group homes over ten years ago. I didn't think that things functioned very well where I worked, I thought that the people living where I worked deserved better than they were offered. I also did find, when starting to study political science, that many of the things happening in the group home had to do with power and politics. So I just started, and then continued, to study the politics of disability, first as a student, then as a doctoral candidate. That's pretty much the story. Now, would you care to present yourselves?
Monica:	Yes we can, you start, Andrea!
Andrea:	I am Andrea. I work with public relations at Grunden. I also work with a project on domestic violence. That's very hush-hush . . . Not everybody have relatives that can help, so it's important. Tomorrow, I am going to Mariestad to lecture for our local organisation about it.
Anders:	I am responsible for the web and our Facebook and our webpage. My name is Anders.
Monica:	I'm Monica. I am staff manager and ombudsman. I work with spreading Grunden to the wider public.
Olof:	My name is Olof and I am the chair of the national organisation of Grunden.
	[One more participant, Emma, will join us later]

In other parts of this book, interview material is presented and directly commented on, thematically sorted, and inserted into a linear argument. This is the regular way of drawing on interviews in social scientific research, a way of writing that ascribes the role of distilling meaning to the researcher. Such narration rests on an epistemological hierarchy that produces texts in which the flow of words of interviewees is continuously interrupted by the textual voice of the scholar. I do not think that this is inherently problematic. However, as the flow of words commented on in this specific chapter deals with representation, it seems necessary to allow the topic of the conversation to influence the way the text is structured. This means that the activists provide material that is treated differently than the interviews with support workers, not because activists with intellectual disability are particularly vulnerable or because I think that this will tear down the hierarchy between us but because the very topic of this chapter concerns the possibilities and limits of a politics of representation.

Monica: I've been working the longest time in Grunden, for 23 years. I have been part of this whole journey. When we started, it was only in Gothenburg, but today we have 19 local organisations.

Niklas: Ok.

Monica: Grunden is unique today. We are working so that people are allowed to take part. We don't want to exclude people, everybody should be welcome. What we do is that we in different ways hire people with disabilities. We have a boss who has a disability. That's what's so special about us. If we go back to 1999, we decided that, ok, we did not want to be part of FUB [The Swedish National Association for Persons with Intellectual Disability]. So, through a long procedure, we decided to be independent. 'How in the world will you be able to handle this . . .?', they were wondering, 'can you do this on your own?' For one year, we dealt with the organisation's economy, hiring people so we didn't have to think about that. Today we do everything else by ourselves. We decide what kind of organisation we want to be. And we have said that to all of our new local organisations: 'you decide!' This has been shocking for many. People like us have never been allowed to decide, but today, we have grown so strong in our organisation that we can make decisions about everything.

Niklas: That's the difference compared to FUB?

Monica: FUB is for the parents, while we represent ourselves.

Andrea: We are really tired of that. Anna Strand started our organisation. She works one floor above us now, at the local organisation of Grunden. She is an honorary member. She realised that when they had board meetings at the time, in FUB, with a mix of disabled and other people, the non-disabled had coffee and buns, whilst the disabled had cookies and soda and balloons. So a lot of stuff like that, those involved at the time were really tired of it. Today, we have a lot of philosophies, like 'participation', we always try to be that. When we are out giving lectures, which I really love doing, it's always those of us with disabilities who give the talks. Not our coaches, because they don't know what it's like to live with an intellectual disability. Nor do those with power over disability politics.

Niklas: I see. Do you cooperate with FUB?

Andrea: Not that much. It's not that we dislike each other, it just hasn't happened that much.

Monica: We have different opinions than they do. But, here in Gothenburg, they've seen that we can handle our organisation, what a success we are. We have some contact with FUB Gothenburg now.

Andrea: I've been working here for 15 years. I couldn't do anything at the start.

Niklas: So, it was challenging?

Andrea: Yes, very much in the beginning. But we learned a lot. If we want to live our lives as everybody else does, then we have to handle it. I have never felt disabled, not ever. My parents told me when I was twelve, but I have never felt it. I have an older brother and they treat me the same as him. So, I didn't feel different. When people say 'you're disabled' I'm like 'uhu, am I?'

At events where I have presented parts of this book, I have been told by fellow scholars that it is crucial that I talk to 'the actual people'. Although I have done so from the start and surely have gained from meeting and knowing people diagnosed with intellectual disability, the suggested reasons for why this is important troubles me. According to my colleagues, the legitimacy of my findings hinges on the support of 'the voice of the intellectually disabled': that 'they' need to be represented and that I have a responsibility to make the 'competent disabled person' visible in my work. In this chapter I speak to people labelled so, but what does engaging the 'voice' of people belonging to this group actually entail? What are the requirements of an 'adequate representation', and why is it precisely 'competency' that should be represented? Is there not a risk that I delimit the possibility to be mediocre, or even bad, at things if I only highlight the over-achieving disabled subject (see Mitchell & Snyder, 2010)?

Hence, there are immediate reasons for caution here. First, it is problematic to presume that there is a unified 'voice' of people with intellectual disabilities, an idea that appears to me as quickly heading towards essentialism. Furthermore, these 'voices' in particular, of the people involved in this particular conversation, all belong to ideologically motivated organised political activists, which most people with intellectual disabilities are not. This is also the case in many projects of 'inclusive research', where activists and scholars collaborate. Hence, there are critical questions to be asked as concerns the underpinnings of my colleagues' calls for representation. The suggestion that I have a responsibility to represent and that the legitimacy of my findings depends on it seems to presume a whole lot about the people belonging to this group. Furthermore, the urge to hear 'the voice' of the intellectually disabled also assumes that these individuals experience the world and the structures of power that they are entangled in only from the viewpoint of their diagnosis but not as inhabiting a certain sex, a certain class, a certain sexual orientation, and a certain race.

These insights mirror the proposition of post-colonial theory that research on disenfranchised groups often tends to attribute to these groups a single and ahistorical consciousness. In Spivak's (1988) analysis of post-colonial patterns of representation, attempts to provide oppressed groups with a 'voice' are bound up with a notion of the subject as coherent, autonomous, and carrying experiences that can be accounted for as 'true' representations of what such people are like (see Varga-Dobai, 2012:2). The role of representatives thus easily becomes to validate and exemplify 'otherness' whilst leaving the very status of being 'other' intact. Focus is directed towards the benevolent and inclusive impulses of the researcher but detracted from how the very idea of a unified identity – be it of people with intellectual disabilities or of the subaltern – itself is an effect of power re-inscribed.

Monica: Eight years ago I was at FUB-Klippan's[2] annual meeting. And we discovered that they had board members without disabilities, who took over proceedings. Like, at one point someone was going to talk, 'no, you are not allowed to talk', this person without disability said. Me and my colleague, sitting at the back, we were only visitors . . . I almost had to put my hand over my colleague's mouth. He was about to boil over.

Niklas: Ok.

Monica: Seeing how people are treated can be horrible. At that board meeting with FUB-Klippan, we had only been there for 10 minutes, everybody was supposed to be 'participating equally', and then we see this. I see how people are treated, at seminars and banquettes and things like that. On these occasions, you often see that personnel, so-called 'normal' staffers, are making fools of themselves. At a conference I attended, I overheard a disabled person wanting to have a beer. All of the seminars for the day were over. And this staffer says 'just so you know, you can only get one'. I just looked, thinking 'Jesus Christ, here I am, sharing a bottle of wine with a colleague', had she heard that I also had a disability, it would have been one hell of a headline . . .

Andrea: Exactly, we can't drink.

Monica: We are not allowed alcohol.

Andrea: They don't know how to handle us.

Monica: Now, how is it for other people? If out on the town, and people are sitting and drinking themselves pissed drunk and become unbearable? That's fine.

Andrea: That's even worse.

Monica: But if we were to be drunk . . .

Andrea: It was like when I was in Jönköping [Swedish town] with Anna. And in the evening, there was supposed to be a party. Only non-alcoholic beer, because they didn't know how to handle us. And I was thinking 'shit . . . what is this?' Later, I was talking to FUB-Klippan, the chair and a non-disabled supporter. And I was talking for an hour about how we are working in Grunden. And suddenly he, the chair of Klippan, said 'but I want to say "developmentally disturbed", rather than 'intellectual disability"'. 'Uhu . . . well say it then'. I don't like the expression, but you can say it. If you say it, then I know. 'But you don't want me to say it', he went on. But I never said that. You can say whatever you like. They even applauded because they wanted to use the term 'developmental disturbance'. I was like, shit, shit, just let them . . . Anna was boiling over. 'Calm down, Anna, calm down'.

Spivak argues (1988) that the impulse to represent, to give voice to, paradoxically mutes: inserting 'the subaltern', or whatever group we seek to represent, into frames of discourse produced from the perspective of the coloniser comprises a form of epistemic violence, where the well-meaning researcher rather than hearing and providing space for the oppressed represents themselves as transparent and as able to give a true account of the authentic needs of the group in question. In her critique of Foucault and Deleuze, targeting this theoretical tendency, Spivak (1988) argues that their accounts are ridden with a troublesome inconsistency as concerns 'the oppressed subject'. While these thinkers generally understand subjectivity as an effect of power, their respective analysis of oppressed groups both presumes the ability of such people to authentically speak for themselves, as 'oppressed', and the capacity of the Western theorist to hear and transparently represent their voices (Spivak, 1988; see Morton, 2003:55). By treating the oppressed subject as singular, Spivak concludes, Foucault's and Deleuze's depictions are in fact constituting this subject whilst concealing their own complicity.

Parallel to this, it seems inherently problematic to account for what people with intellectual disabilities are like, rendered so by the general discourse within which I am supposed to make their voices heard. In disability studies, there has been an on-going discussion about non-disabled researchers who write about disability and about the need to include people with disabilities in research (see Barnes, 1996; Chappel, 2000; Barnes, 2003; Walmsley, 2004; McClimens, 2007). 'Nothing about us without us', the slogan of the disability movement goes. There is a hidden presumption underpinning this slogan, namely that there is equivalence between the two 'us'; that nothing *about* people with disability, the general group, ought to be said without the involvement of specific people from this group.[3] As not *all* people with disability, for practical reasons, can participate in research, the notion of representation is implicit.

Here, it is relevant to ponder Butler's (1990:3) suggestion that the designation of 'women' as the subject of feminism itself is a discursive formation of representational politics which can be assumed to re-inscribe domination on the subject position which is supposed to be emancipated. Are there not similar risks associated with designating 'the intellectually disabled subject' to be the agent of emancipatory research or of emancipation-through-representation more generally? Although I strongly advocate the inclusion of people with intellectual disabilities in research, caution is needed – as concerns using specific individuals to represent 'intellectual disability' and as concerns representing people of this group as a unified political agent.

Monica: We have all of these things to deal with. That is what makes us unique. It is Emma, Olof, Andrea, and me and we are a group of people living in danger. Our disabilities are invisible. We speak for ourselves, we have a politician among us,[4] and we have developed during these years. If we go back to 2009 when the national organisation of Grunden was established, then we didn't know what the platform would look like. Today, we have an employed boss with disability, who also takes care of all the tough things coming along, the things that all other bosses take care of, with contracts and all of that, and who takes charge when difficult situations come up. You have done that.

Olof: Yes . . .
Monica: If this were 10 or 15 years ago, people would have been like 'Olof, you will not manage this . . .', but now you are at all of these meetings and you handle it.
Olof: Yes, I guess I do.
Niklas: Would you like to tell us a little bit about this?
Olof: Sometimes I sit with the National Board of Health and Welfare [Swe: Socialstyrelsen]. I have even been to meetings with IVO [the Swedish Supervisory Authority of Health and Welfare].
Niklas: Ok . . .
Olof: I mean, something like that . . . I had the hunch that they would be shocked. They don't notice that I am disabled, because it's not something you can see. I bet they would scratch their heads and think 'something is not right here . . .' if they knew. In that way, we have really crushed the myth that 'people with disabilities, what can they do?'
Monica: As staff manager, I take courses in order to become better. A few years ago, they would have sent a coach with me who would function as an interpreter . . . 'is everything ok . . . are you managing . . .?' But it was as easy as anything.
Andrea: Before we got our own organisation, it was always the staff working with us that went. They attended these courses, it was 'them' and 'us'. We don't want that.

The voice of people with intellectual disabilities, like the voice of 'the worker' or of the 'subaltern', often appears to be represented by a political proxy standing in as the 'voice' of the group in question. When people suggest to me that I must include interviews with people with intellectual disabilities, it seems to be underpinned by precisely such a mythology of 'the voice'; a 'voice' that can validate, not by providing important information or strengthening my argument but by standing in as the very category itself. By *being* intellectual disability. Ellis (2014:494) notes that the energies mobilised to describe 'otherness' in the most authentic way possible seem to be a search for lost origins. The idea that the 'voice' of people with intellectual disabilities provides legitimacy to my arguments can therefore be understood against the backdrop of a modernist drive to access the centre, the core, the essence of whatever we seek to understand (see Ellis, 2014:502). Indeed, modernist traces of representation permeate projects of emancipation, privileging 'presence' codified as what is spoken and made explicit. The inquiries of colleagues who wonder whether I aim to speak to 'the actual people' connect to this trope of representational thinking.

Emma: Hi! I am very interested in these things, can I say something?
Niklas: Yes, of . . .
Emma: [interrupts] You, who are a researcher and all, why does it still say 'developmental disturbance' in the LSS? Why do you 'compli-velopmentally disturbed' [sve: 'invecklingsstörda'] not have your own law, when it is you that complicates matters with all your laws and paragraphs?

Niklas: Well . . .
Emma: . . . Whilst we try to develop society.
Niklas: We can talk about that. We talked about that [on the phone, with Monica, when arranging the meeting], about the terminology of 'developmental disturbance', why is this a bad word?
Andrea: I can tell you that. It started with Anna [Strand, founder of Grunden], you can see that she has [a disability], because she's got Down syndrome. In Grunden, we don't judge based on diagnoses, we see each other as people instead. We don't care about that, we want to live as others, in society. We want to be people. We don't want to be filed under labels. They called me from Eskilstuna [Swedish city], 'I am going now, to meet staff and "service-users" ', they said, 'I am sorry, but you mean "people", not "users"!' They never called back.
Niklas: Ok . . .
Andrea: It says 'developmentally disturbed' in the law . . . When I moved to a new apartment within Gothenburg, they had to write down that I was 'developmentally disturbed'. So I said 'can you write at the margins that I am not developmentally disturbed, that I am Andrea?'. 'No, I can't', they responded. 'Well, you have to or I leave here and now. It's your choice', I said.
Niklas: What did they do?
Andrea: She had to write it. Because I am not only helping myself, I am also helping those who cannot speak for themselves.

Grunden is the first organisation in Sweden 'of' rather than 'for' people with intellectual disabilities. Its function is described as being a platform for members of this group to represent themselves. Hence, there is a considerable degree of transgression of pre-established expectations here, relating to what Simons (1995:103) calls '[a] politics of those who refuse to be what they are and strive to become other'. Historically, self-advocacy of people with this diagnosis has been rare, as the political movement of intellectual disability rights has been dominated by a number of organisations ruled by parents and relatives, at least in Sweden. Consequently, representing oneself goes beyond the activists speaking for themselves. It also means that they are portraying themselves as subjects that are capable of acting politically. Demanding to be called by name – 'Andrea'! – rather than by diagnosis thus becomes a subversive action. In this sense, two aspects of 'representation' are operating in tandem: representation as 'speaking for', as in political representation, and as 'depicting' oneself as a political agent.

Niklas: You were about to say something, Emma . . .?
Emma: I was going to say that all people develop, but what does 'disturbance' mean?
Andrea: Yes!
Monica: That's right.
Emma: The word 'disturbance' is not in our dictionary. And as regards people that need supported living, if someone on the staff says that they are

going to Pelle [a generic Swedish name], then they usually say 'I'm going to the "user" . . .' Why can't they say 'I'm going to the tenant'? We have the same right to our apartments as you, who are 'compli-velopmentally' disturbed. I have gotten the City of Gothenburg to investigate whether people attending day-care services can get salary rather than 'activity benefits'.[5] For many of us, like Andrea or me, where you can't see the disability – we often fall between the chairs. Social insurance says that we are too healthy to receive sick insurance, whilst the job centre say that we can't work because we are disabled. And because of the law on day-care services, we can't go to the job centre activities, so we can't get social insurance. What would you do?

Niklas: I don't know. I mean . . . I guess I think that if you work, you should get paid properly for it. Activity benefits, I mean . . . I know people that work just like anybody else, just as good as anybody else does, but since you do it as disabled, getting it as a service rather than as a job, you don't get paid properly. To me, that is injustice.

Emma: I have gotten the municipality, here in Gothenburg, the board of adult schooling and the board of labour market issues, they want to have a discussion with us at Grunden to change the system. Here, in Gothen-burg, they have taken away Fas 3 [phase 3],[6] this is the next step, maybe.

There are so many ideas about intellectual disability coming into conflict with the activists' own conceptions of who they are. In our conversation, they often refer to the stupidity of such ideas. The fact that it is possible to provide these stories as examples of narrow-mindedness and prejudice, to mock them and laugh at them, indicates both an awareness of the norms that dictate how their diagnosis is seen and a position from where it is possible to scrutinise these norms. But, in parallel to Butler's (2005) line of reasoning, it is nevertheless in relation to these norms that subject formation becomes possible, even when resisted. The organ-isational context of Grunden seems to be a space in which these stories can be told and in which subjectivities can be articulated in contention with dominating ideas on intellectual disability. However, it is not a space where popular discourse about intellectual disability is absent. To the contrary, it seems to be continuously talked about, referred to, and questioned. The biopolitical constitution of intellectual dis-ability, limiting and damaging as it is described in the conversation, is both the target and the necessary precondition of the activist's resistance.

Andrea: It's like, when you are disabled . . . I got LSS when I was 7, because I was too young to decide. I can accept that. But, I did not get to decide that, so I got a label on my forehead that I am good for nothing. I want to work out there, on the market . . .

Niklas: The labour market?

Andrea: Yes. But I have other problems, like a hearing impairment. But I have had got to prove it. I have been an intern in child care, because I love kids. So, I went out and I had to prove it. It's like a label on my forehead that I am developmentally disturbed, and it's there because of the legislation.

Niklas: How do you do that? You know, because it seems like one of the things your organisation wants to do is to discard that label on the forehead . . .

Monica: What we do, and that's why we are unique, and I had been at day-care centres for 17 years, and 5 years ago, I became employed instead. At the start, I was kind of proud that I had reached that point, to get paid. But it's a whole lot of work before that. I have no guarantees, if I lose my job, I am outside the service-system, and then I have to apply again. As things look today, things can go very badly for me.

Niklas: One thing I am thinking is that there is one set of rules for, well, people like me, who are not . . .

Emma: Who are compli-velopmentally disturbed!

Niklas: Yeah, if you are 'compli-velopmentally disturbed', then you can do lots of stupid stuff. You know, I've been to group homes where you're not allowed to have more than three cups of coffee a day. Some support workers that I've interviewed tell me this while having three cups just over the duration of my interview. So there are different standards.

Monica: I have been living in group homes. At one point, I was having shrimp and wine with my boyfriend on a Wednesday. All of a sudden, a staffer just enters the apartment, for some stupid reason, they wanted to borrow a whiteboard pencil, she said. And I don't have one. It was only that they wanted to check . . . you know, how things work. I had windows in my apartment.

Andrea: If you were drunk or something?

Monica: Or if I was doing something naughty with my boyfriend.

During a few instances in the conversation, Emma addresses me by referring to my status of not being intellectually disabled; 'you, the researcher'; 'the compli-velopmentally disturbed'; and so on. Interestingly, she invokes this as a rhetorical gesture when drawing attention to something she finds strange and unjust. During these instances, such strangeness becomes associated with me, and there is a clear sense of the dividing line between 'norm' and 'deviance' being re-inscribed, as well as an awareness of the distribution of power which comes out of it. By pointing towards this line, however, something happens to the hierarchy of the relationship. I represent the categorisation, the distinction between us that she seeks to challenge, and she does so by naming my 'normalcy'. This works to undermine my pre-established authority; it contests the culturally held presumption that researchers know something while people with intellectual disabilities know nothing.

Andrea: Excuse me . . .

Niklas: Go ahead!

Andrea: Always when I lecture, I say 'I am not disabled, I am societally disabled'. It is society that made me so. I have never felt disabled, not in my whole life. It's society. So, I have never had that problem. I am going to Mariestad tomorrow and I will say that again.

Niklas: If you see yourself as impaired, then you go to the doctor or to rehab. But if you see yourself as 'socially disabled', then you become a member of Grunden . . .?

Andrea: That's why we are doing this, to change things.

Niklas: So, somehow attitudes . . .

Andrea: Yes, the attitudes in society aren't good. Let's say I go by the tram or something, if you walk strange or something, as some friends of mine do, then people stare. 'Is something wrong?' I say to those looking. I am not afraid to do that, to speak my mind. One time, in the grocery store, someone was really staring at me. I was thinking 'ok, what's wrong now . . .?' She really glared at me. When I left, do you know what I said? 'Go buy a TV if you want something to stare at!' She really panicked. I know that it was not nice, but I could not help it.

Niklas: I can see that one becomes fed up.

Andrea: Yes, you really do get fed up. I am only human, there's a limit to how much I can take.

The displacement of taken-for-granted role ascriptions is also evident in the terminological invention of 'compli-velopmental disturbance'. The term is an intricate word play, alluding to the fact that the antonym of 'develop' in Swedish is the same word as 'complicate'. Thus, this inversion of 'developmental disturbance' that Emma uses as a label for 'normal' people literally means having a disturbance of complicating matters. It operates by attaching to normalcy, to the 'compli-velopmentally disturbed', a kind of deficit that mirrors 'developmental disturbance'. When first introducing the specific term, Emma explicitly stated that it was 'us', the 'compli-velopmentally disturbed', who complicated matters infinitely, with special laws and regulations that do not make sense. As such, this way of addressing normalcy interrupts how otherness is articulated within the hegemonic discourse. Through the use of 'compli-velopmental disturbance', Emma raises questions concerning whose standpoint should be the voice of 'reason' and whose mode of address should be privileged.

Emma: It was a few years ago, a TV show about Glada Huddik [a theatre group famous for having intellectually disabled actors], Per Johansson, their boss, was there in the TV studio. Do you know what I said?

Niklas: No.

Emma: I said 'you put us with disabilities in a cage like monkeys and feed us bananas. But we are humans that need just as much love as anybody, we are not small monkeys in a cage!'

Niklas: Yeah, I've also been thinking about this show *En annan del av Köping* [Swedish documentary series about life in a group home, Eng: *Another Part of Köping*] . . .

Andrea: Oh my god.

Olof: I was watching half a show or something like that, and I turned it off thinking what kind of degrading kind of thing is this . . .

Andrea: They do not tell stories about real lives. It's only cuteness and all nice . . . It's like everybody with intellectual disabilities likes dance band music [a genre which has been subjected to much mockery due to its low-brow status in Sweden] and hugging. What's that all about?

Monica: I was on *SVT Debatt* [Swedish weekly television show hosting debates on topical issues] one and a half months ago. With Olof. I was so pissed off, because there were professors there, doctors, who are supposed to be so smart and good. I couldn't keep quiet, so I raised my hand and said 'We live in the 21st century, I am a mother, I have an intellectual disability, if we were not here, how would the world be?' The debate was about prenatal diagnosis.

Niklas: That's also something I'd like to talk about . . .

Monica: You can watch the show.

Niklas: Yes, I watched it.

Emma: What was your name again?

Niklas: Niklas Altermark.

Emma: I have no idea when it comes to names.

Niklas: As a matter of fact I have a friend who said that I would probably meet you, he is a member of the same political party as you here in Gothenburg.

Emma: It is funny that you say that, it highlights that we can do things like that.

Niklas: Perhaps it's like with *SVT Debatt*. It isn't always the professors and medical professionals who have the smartest views.

Andrea: Ann, who was here earlier [a woman entered to ask something earlier during the conversation], she wanted to say something in the studio, but didn't get a chance. Later, we learned that she was only there to show what Down syndrome looks like.

All: What!?

Andrea: Yes, Erik and I were told that. They wanted to show Down syndrome . . . what about that?

Monica: Now, I am even more pissed off.

Throughout our talk, tensions arose in relation to the construction of the 'intellectually disabled citizen' of Swedish disability politics. It appears that most of the activists do not view themselves as supporters of the present legislation of citizenship inclusion. On the other hand, the language of the politics of inclusion frames their political agency and therefore provides them with a terminology to parse political demands. This exemplifies the intertwined nature of flows of power and practices of resistance; their contestation of the present order of things is formulated in the dominant humanist and liberal vocabulary, yet its meaning is recurrently shifted. They demand 'citizenship', albeit a lack of belief in the legislation granting them precisely that; although 'participation', 'rights', and 'living as others' play a large part in the conversation, here this vocabulary is used to name an ideal which lies ahead, in the future, rather than in the policy texts that were supposed to provide for their emancipation. Hence, the activists are making up their own script by shifts and disruptions internal to the existing one, creating their own conditions of possibility, but *within* the established language of post-institutionalisation. In our conversation, it seems that we are searching for a political alternative that lies beyond the language at our disposal and, in a sense, this alternative presents itself as performed rather than fully articulated.

Niklas: I believe many think that, no matter what it is with you, it must be the disability . . . ache in the ears or the foot, depressed . . . As soon as something arises, then it is explained by disability. It reduces you to a diagnosis. What do you think about this? What can you do about it?

Emma: Lecture . . . as we are doing with you! Then you can write a book about it that may lead to something. Throw away all the old books. Throw away the old books, write new ones. I became disabled when I was six. I was out walking in the woods with my little brother and Daddy, who walked in front of us. My brother shouted 'Dad, I can't wake Emma up'. In the ambulance, they said that they should be prepared that I would not make it. When they realised that I would, they said that I would be a 'vegetable' for the rest of my life, I would not be able to learn how to sit, to walk, to talk . . . But what am I doing today? I am speaking and I am a politician.

Andrea: Thank God for that, say your parents . . .

Emma: In 2012, I became a politician, just like that. Even though I am disabled, I can talk. When you meet rehab personnel or group home staff . . . some think that we can't talk for ourselves. So, you have to have someone speaking for you who follows you around all the time.

Andrea: Yes, I was also supposed to have this kind of woman with me. Then she quit. And my case worker became fixated on this. She was rude to me. When we had a meeting, I said, 'I think you weren't very nice to me'. And I like to look people in the eyes when I speak. And then she became really uneasy. That was her way of saying that people with disabilities, we should always obey . . .

Emma: . . . follow orders.

Again, there is a reversal of roles as Emma declares that they are lecturing me. I am not there to hear and represent them, nor for the benefit of my research. Rather, Emma suggests that they see my visit in instrumental terms, where they are using me to amplify and promote their viewpoints. Since I have been educated in social science, still somewhat under the spell of the idea of the objective researcher, this instils some uneasiness: what does it mean for the validity of my material if the interviewees are motivated by political strategy?

Pillow (2003 in Varga-Dobai, 2012:9) has argued for a 'reflexivity of discomfort' as concerns the relationship between researcher and research subjects. Such a reflexivity renders the relationships between the knowing Self and those being researched tenuous and troubling. This corresponds to how I experience our talk, in which I am surprised, questioned, and made accountable for the hierarchical relationship between people with intellectual disabilities and 'normal' people. Importantly, the stimulus for this comes from them rather than from my meta-theoretical presuppositions, especially in those instances when they make explicit that there is a divide separating us. They address me as distinct from what they are, no matter our mutual awareness of my personal sympathy and alliance with their cause. Paradoxically, this has the effect of making me question the meaning of the lines of demarcations as such. It urges me to start to ask questions about whether it is possible to establish a mode of conversation of speaking *with* rather than *about* people made 'other', and if sometimes this could be an issue of *them* forcing *me* to hear what they have to say rather than me acting as a good listener.

Emma: Niklas, I have made a lot of proposals for our party congress. And I am disabled. I am not supposed to be able to do that, but I have – about tobacco, special schooling, and lots of other things. And I am 'developmentally disturbed'. But I can write all of these things anyway. I have written lots of debate articles, if you Google me and search for my name you will find lots of articles I have written. And I am supposed to know nothing, I can't even make my own tea. [. . .] I am better at dragging politicians here. The first year we had the Social Policy Committee from the national parliament visiting us. The second year, I invited politicians from the Committee of Education. The third year I invited the Committee of the Labour Market. This year we had guests from the Committee of Social Insurance. If you look at Mickel or Johnny [two, provided the context of the talk, supposedly non-disabled persons occupying the room next door], they would never manage that.

Niklas: That's how I think, too. We are good at different things. I am good at cooking, my fiancée can't . . .

Monica: . . . That's how it's like for us too, I am the chef at our place because I have problems with my eyes, so I can't do other stuff needed to be done at home.

Niklas: . . . but some of these things, that you can be less good at . . . they are bundled together and labelled 'intellectual disability'. I think that everybody should get support if they need, but within the group of people called 'disabled' there are too many needs to name them all.

Monica: Ok, I am sorry, but I got to leave now. Here is a t-shirt for you, since you've been so nice and come here. And here is our magazine that you can read on the train. Promote us in Lund [the city of the university where I was working at the time]!

Niklas: Yes, it has been so great to talk to you.

Monica: Normally, we charge people for this, but today you get it for free . . .

Niklas: Thanks.

Monica: It's part of our job. It's how we make a living.

Andrea: I would not survive without it.

    [Monica leaves]

Emma: I have a question for you. You are a researcher, or whatever you are . . .

Niklas: Yeah.

Emma: In the first paragraph of the UN declaration, it says that all people, also according to the convention of the rights of children, that all have the same rights. But since the law of special schooling is older than the law of discrimination, the law of discrimination cannot interfere when kids in special schooling don't get equal grades. But kids in special schools should have a right to equal grades. UN says that all have equal rights, but if a compli-mentally disturbed kid is wrongly placed in a special school, then they get compensation. If a person with a disability is placed in special schools, they don't, never mind that they are just transferred to day-care after graduation, rather than the labour market. Since we get day-care, and aren't prepared for working, we cannot earn money to get good pensions. We have many people working as cleaners within day-care, but they are not allowed to enter the unions.

Niklas: Yes, I agree about this difference, also Swedish disability policy is . . .

Emma: That's what I am trying to change.

Niklas: Yes . . .

Emma: That's why I do all of these things.

In the words of Wisweswaran (1994 in Varga-Dobai, 2012:12), one way to formulate the broader purpose of this chapter is as searching for a self-reflexive research practice of 'betrayal', deliberately questioning its own authority to represent. When repressing the impulse to unify, clarify, and explain the meaning of the voices of people with intellectual disabilities into an overriding and homogenous argument, there may be a mode of analysis that allows the researcher to be surprised, hence forcing me to reflect on my own presumptions.

In Spivak's work, the subaltern is speechless due to the colonial inability of heeding their voices. In this conversation, the activists are forcing me to listen. Theoretically, I have not assumed their inability to exercise this kind of agency. Yet in the context of analysing this conversation, it is striking how discursive features of their address change the framing of the talk and how that makes me lose my train of thought and preconceived ideas of what my analytical purpose is. If the inability of the dispossessed to speak stems from their inability to be heard, I would suggest that no discourse is so firm that it renders impossible resistance by means of discursive shifts that force the dominant party to learn how to listen. In this context, resistance seems to be the practice of forcing non-disabled individuals to unlearn their inability to acknowledge the viewpoints of people with intellectual disabilities.

Niklas: As I see it, the law is really clear that in group homes, locked doors are not allowed, tenants have the right to come and go as they wish. It's not a prison.

Emma: They say 'risk of fire'.

Niklas: Risk of fire?

Emma: Yes, they use that. But we have the same right to risk burning down our homes as anybody. As any compli-velopmentallally disturbed. I have invented that word.

Niklas: Yes, I figured.

Emma: Since I am also a politician, I feel that . . . why don't you have your own law? We are all under the general social care law, why isn't it so that LSS helps those in need? When it really matters, the case workers break the law. The LSS says that with day-care services, as far as possible the individual should decide where she wants to work, but case workers don't care about that. They just go, 'you should be there and you should be there and you should be there!' But if I want to be over there instead . . .? 'No, you should go there!' You are not allowed to have a bottle of red any day because you can't take care of yourself. But your mother doesn't call you [directed at me] to ask 'are you drunk?'

Niklas: No.

It follows from Spivak's argument that the oppressed has no place other than as 'spoken for' within the dominating discourse. The possibility to understand 'the other' is circumscribed by the discourses that we have at our disposal, precisely since there can be no knowledge of otherness outside a language that renders certain subjects 'other' (Kapoor, 2004:636). To represent oneself also means to re-present oneself as a political agent, against the designation of otherness and speechlessness.

In light of this, the accounts provided by the activists of their refusal of derogatory terms such as 'developmental disturbance' also seem to be a refusal to accept the linguistic and epistemological conditions of their emergence. As Goodley (2014:xi) has noted, (intellectual) disability is all too often immediately linked to pathology, marked by a set of medical terms that are assumed to be neutral. The activists displace this linkage by forming new conceptual constellations, for example linking together 'disability' with 'contestation', 'intellectual disability' with 'self-representation', and by questioning the division between 'disability' and 'normalcy'. One way to read Spivak on 'postcolonialism' is as a reminder that our representation can never escape the bias of our positioning (see Kapoor, 2004). My way of seeing this conversation is that resistance may present itself in instances when the speech of groups rendered 'other' unsettle such bias, making it visible and exposing its limits.

Notes

1 Apart from this main theme, I also raised a set of questions that specifically focused on experiences of LSS services, which was referred to in Chapter 5. These parts of our conversation will not be presented here.
2 A branch of FUB specifically for people with intellectual disabilities.
3 Here, I am indebted to the stimulating feedback of Katarina Jacobsson on a previous paper.
4 Emma, yet to arrive, is an elected official in local government.
5 'Activity benefits' are paid to individuals granted day-care service.
6 Fas3 was a Swedish unemployment program which forced individuals who have been unemployed for a certain amount of time to work unpaid in order to get social insurance. The program has been widely criticised as a prime example of neoliberal 'workfare' politics.

8 Ethics

There are two reasons for ending this book with a chapter on prenatal diagnosis. First, as the practices of scanning for certain conditions are underpinned by judgements of pathology and hence can be seen as an expression of biopolitics, the subsequent examination summarises and ties together many of the themes that have been discussed throughout the book. Second, as resistance against prenatal diagnosis is often embedded in discourses of 'ethics', examining how present scanning practices are understood and fought against can serve as a bridge into a concluding discussion on the overarching ethos of my own research project and on the possibility of mobilising an ethics of resistance. Thus, this is not another attempt at criticising prenatal diagnosis, as there have been many of, but an attempt to critically discuss the discursive limits of the resistance against prenatal diagnosis.

In the two previous chapters, I have argued that resistance is pertinent in situations in which the inclusive and exclusive aspects of the government of intellectual disability comes into friction. Yet the emergence of resistance is necessarily preconditioned by the prevailing mode of government, and, therefore, contestations may end up strengthening the particular order that is contested, as when 'care' is mobilised to legitimate paternalism or when self-representation turns into essentialism. This also holds for attempts to resist the present organisation of prenatal screening. Accordingly, there are numerous attempts, by disability organisations and disability scholars, to critically assess and sometimes question screening practices. I will argue that these are hampered by how this is understood as an 'ethical' rather than a 'political' question. This has the troubling consequence that the political rationales of prenatal diagnosis are obscured in favour of moralisation and individualisation, where prenatal diagnosis is deceitfully de-politicised because moral arguments take precedence over analyses of power.

In what follows, against the 'ethical' framing and in order to re-politicise the issue, I will argue that we need to acknowledge how practices of prenatal screening are technologies of government and that this very insight provide an opportunity to re-politicise ethics, urging us to rethink the fundamentals of the government of intellectual disability in light of critique as an ethical stance towards oneself and others.

Ethics as 'resistance without politics'

Some five years ago I met a person diagnosed with Down syndrome wearing a T-shirt that said 'Jag är utrotningshotad' (*Eng:* 'I am under threat of extinction'). The message, of course, referred to the increased use of prenatal testing, which has resulted in growing numbers of pregnancies being terminated due to conditions associated with intellectual disability. The message struck me as peculiar; it operates by inserting 'Down syndrome', the phenomenon, into a discourse associated with endangered animals, however, underhandedly insisting precisely that people with Down syndrome are *not* animals, as if the subtext read 'you are endangering my kind as if I were an animal, but you won't notice or admit it'. Hence, the T-shirt text highlighted the conflict that exists between policy promises of equal value and the actual practices of erasure. In my gut, that T-shirt made me realise that the issue at stake here is that, sometimes, only certain lives are considered worth living. In this sense, prenatal diagnosis actualises Butler's (1993:xiii) fundamental question concerning which human beings are allowed to become subjects, worthy of grievance and worthy of protection (see Samuels, 2002:60).

As prenatal screening has become obstetrical practice in many countries, questions have been raised concerning how this will affect attitudes towards people living with disabilities and what the world will lose when certain syndromes are disappearing. These discussions are now taking place in light of new non-invasive tests being introduced into the growing market of pregnancy management, tests which only require small samples of maternal blood to provide allegedly conclusive results. These are cheap, safe, and easy to use, which means that it is likely that they will further reduce the number of births of people with Down syndrome and other conditions associated with intellectual disability (Kaposy, 2013:299).[1] As with the introduction of other screening techniques, the new tests have caused debate and worries within the disability movement. At the same time, however, they appear hard to fight against. Influential disability organisations regularly work to create more positive images of intellectual disability and to inform parents about support systems and the right to choose, however, rarely targeting the politics of screening itself. Hence, these organisations have primarily sought to point out the fact that people born with Down syndrome today can live rich and meaningful lives without really calling for such tests to be abandoned or for the state to prevent their use. As I will argue, this is typical and a consequence of how prenatal screening is discursively framed as an issue of 'ethics', which delimits what becomes possible to say and think about the issue. Before turning to develop this argument, however, we must first look into some fundamentals of prenatal testing.

Practices of screening

Modern scanning technologies equip us with the ability to, more or less, eliminate a number of syndromes associated with intellectual disability. While working on this book, I have met quite a few people who are seriously concerned that this will happen in many countries within the foreseeable future.[2] The procedures surrounding prenatal diagnosis differ considerably between and within states (see Buckley & Buckley, 2008:79; EUROCAT, 2010): some recommend screening all pregnant women, combining it with more or less explicit incentives and recommendations that affected pregnancies should be terminated, whilst other countries set an age for when testing is offered, most often at a maternal age of 35. What more or less all programs of prenatal testing have in common, which will be key to my analysis, is that the coercive force of the state is absent: health care and maternal care provide information, sometimes strong recommendations, but parents decide (see EUROCAT, 2010).

Prenatal diagnosis starts with an initial screening that provides a probability calculation measuring the likelihood of a set of medically defined conditions (Vanstone & Kinsella, 2010:453). The purpose of the initial screening is to estimate whether it is necessary to go through with invasive and conclusive testing, which presents further risks for the foetus. This means that there is a cutoff point (usually at the point where the probability of having an affected baby exceeds the risk of hurting the foetus by testing) for when it is recommended that one follows through with amniocentesis (Buckley & Buckley, 2008:79). In turn, programs of prenatal testing must balance the detection rate with the risks associated with invasive testing. The significance of the new non-invasive blood tests is that they take this balancing of 'risks' and 'benefits' out of the equation; there will be no need to refrain from testing out of concerns for the safety of the foetus.

There are different reports on the effects of prenatal diagnosis on the overall number of people with syndromes screened for. On the one hand, increasing maternity age of parents in many countries means that the effect of prenatal diagnosis is hampered since the likelihood of having children with Down syndrome increases with maternal age (see Buckley & Buckley, 2008:79). What can be said with certainty is that prenatal diagnosis significantly diminishes the relative number of births of children with syndromes associated with intellectual disability; in most contexts, termination rates of affected pregnancies range from 65 to 90% (see Mansfield et al., 1999; Buckley & Buckley, 2008; Kaposy, 2013). Hence, prenatal diagnosis appears to be a highly efficient means of decreasing the number of certain kinds of human beings entering the world.

'Ethicisation'

Now, a striking feature of how testing practices are publicly discussed and academically analysed is the focus on moral imperatives. Hence, there are on-going debates concerning whether prenatal testing and the termination of some pregnancies can be justified, on what grounds, and given what premises. It is also within this discourse that we find many of the objections to contemporary testing, in which disability scholars, along with representatives of the disability movement, question the justifications of today's practices (Amundson & Tresky, 2007; Kaposy, 2013). This debate has gained some popular recognition, as utilitarian philosophers such as Peter Singer (1993) and Jeff McMahan (1996) (in)famously argue for the termination of pregnancies that will result in disabled lives and in which Singer even argues that killing disabled infants can be justified. Naturally, this has caused a moral philosophical trench war with representatives and advocates of the disability movement. The arguments proposed by disability advocates are often geared to appeal to our moral sentiments, where principles of rights to exist, to equal human dignity, and the like are proposed as presenting a case for the preservation of human diversity (see Parens & Asch, 2003; Kaposy, 2013). This can be read as a neat illustration of how resistance is discursively pre-structured: with the 'ethicisation' of prenatal testing follows an 'ethicised' resistance, and thereby a framework of ethics comes to compose the main battlefield over prenatal diagnosis. An exemplary case of this ethical framing can be seen in Shakespeare (2006:85–102): whereas *Disability Rights and Wrongs* essentially is a book about disability and social theory, the issue of prenatal diagnosis is solely discussed in terms of moral justification and moral philosophy without ever coming close to an analysis of power. As I will argue, the possibility that there are other issues, outside the scope of 'what can be justified?' which may be of equal or even greater importance than moral justifications, has been lost along the way. Of course, issues of power are occasionally pointed out by disability scholars and advocates (see Parens & Asch, 2012, for an overview), but, even in those cases, they are rarely developed into a proper analysis of government.

There are two sides to the ethical framing. On the one hand, as discussed, it leads to philosophical arguments concerning which decisions are possible to justify (see Singer, 1993; Heyd, 1995; Shakespeare, 2006; Amundson & Tresky, 2007; Kaposy, 2013). On the other hand, it also seems to suggest that prenatal diagnosis pertains to individual decisions that politics has no business interfering in (see García et al., 2008). At least in Europe, critical voices of disability organisations have most often refused to side with the anti-abortion movement, to their credit, staunchly refraining from moralising on individual choices. But as the ethical questions regarding prenatal diagnosis are interpreted as primarily concerning expecting individuals, there is no obvious arena left to be politicised. As an effect of the ethical framing, the rationales of individual parents seem to be the only possible target of resistance, which on the other hand makes the issue appear as being about abortion and the right to choose. By extension, many disability organisations mobilise to provide pregnant people with better and more nuanced information to base their judgement on. However, this mode of resistance reifies the individualised framing of the issue. As such, issues pertaining to power, to discursive constructions of the diagnoses targeted, and to societal and cultural attitudes rarely enter public discussion on prenatal diagnosis – among neither its advocates nor its opponents. The frequent returns to the personal and individual nature of these choices in the literature on prenatal testing reinforces the impression that the aggregate effects of screening are regarded as beside the point (Acharya, 2011:30; García et al., 2008; Addington & Rapoport, 2012:513; Skirton et al., 2014).

The ethical framework has been further strengthened by the rise of bioethics as an academic field of research. The underlying narrative of this discipline is that technological and scientific advances give rise to new ethical dilemmas (Vailly, 2008:2541), whilst at the same time continuously leaving out the societal attitudes and drivers of these technological advancements. Intuitively, this perspective may seem appealing: first, it is a call for caution against the un-reflected use of scientific innovations and, second, it urges us to consider these innovations in light of moral questions which had previously been rarely considered in debates about policy and science. However, as Amundson and Tresky (2007:541–2) note, what becomes an issue of bioethics in the first place is far from evident. The bioethical debates about 'disability' are primarily preoccupied with questions about the conditions that make it morally permissible to end or prevent disabled lives (see Wolbring, 2003). This should make us suspicious. Why ask these questions? What circumstances must be in place for such questions to be asked? What questions are concurrently suspended? Not surprisingly, people with disabilities are notably absent from these discussions (see Wolbring, 2003:175).

'Ethics' as an effect of politics

Now, to understand what this way of discussing prenatal diagnosis entails, I contend that it is necessary to examine what it excludes.

The question of practical ethics in the context of prenatal diagnosis is 'what can be justified?' The question of politics, to the contrary (and as I deploy this notoriously abstract concept), is 'how does power operate?' It follows that when an issue is framed as 'ethical', our focus is detracted from asking questions concerning how our views are shaped, by what actors, and to what means, in favour of questions regarding what views can be justified, by what arguments, and to what assumingly universal moral end (see Brown, 2008:109–10). This means that many of the theoretical tools we associate with political action and activism are rendered out of bounds in discussions about prenatal diagnosis. In order to productively engage with and resist the present order of things, it is necessary to instead consider what is happening when biopolitics is made into a question of ethics in the first place, that is, to study 'the ethical question' as a political effect rather than as an ethical problem to be solved.

First, as hinted at already, the discourse of ethics has the effect of *individualising* prenatal diagnosis. How should parents act? How should the state provide parents with information to act on? Do individuals who have suffered from a 'wrongful birth' have a legitimate claim to compensation? Do their parents (see Pritchard, 2005)? Provided this way of asking questions, bioethicists are made authorities on dilemmas facing individual parents, providing them with grounds for justification but never shedding light on the underlying power relations between disabled and non-disabled people. It is a distinctively liberal framing, where everything revolves around the choices of individuals. Underpinning the ethicisation of prenatal testing is the view that it presents parents with a 'moral or existential dilemma', as Kelly (2009:82) formulates it, or that it constitutes a 'very personal decision', as Addington and Rapoport (2012:513) have it. These formulations are indicative of how the macro-politics of technological and scientific advances are transformed into individual quandaries. When we ask 'the ethical question' in this way, we mask the political stakes of knowledge and technology, instead pushing individuals to solve conflicts of power through personal ethical investiture.

A second limitation coming out of this discourse concerns how the ethical framework obscures our understanding of *government* by depicting the relationship between the state and morals as a matter of choosing sound principles. Rather than asking how power operates, we are asking how power can be justified. Thus, as long as the state acts by sensible doctrines, and as long as prenatal diagnosis is coupled with balanced information and the informed consent of parents, as many bioethicists would have it, we can be assured that there is no need for criticism and that everything is working out fine (see Acharya, 2011:30; Skirton et al., 2014). This conceptualisation of the relationship between state and ethics rests on a moral universalism, which holds that certain principles transcend the messy world of politics, although this messy world should ideally be guided by such universal principles. This presumption means that the complexity of government is not sufficiently handled and that power, culture, and discourse are implicitly seen as hindrances to detecting moral truths. In the context of bioethics, power relations, discourses, and subject formation are all discarded when ethical guidance for testing procedures are being derived. As a result, the ways that parents are understood to make these choices in the bioethical literature ends up being a complete fiction, since the depiction of the decision-making process ignores the ways that subjects are *always* entangled in relationships of power and acting in context. Thus, how parents carry cultural presumptions about intellectual disability and how they are targeted by biased or unbiased information, are regarded as distractions from the question of how the state ought to perform screening.

Resistance that takes the ethical framing for granted will consequently continue to obscure the way that power is exercised. What we get can be characterised as 'resistance without politics', a kind of oscillation between seeking to convince would-be parents that they should not terminate pregnancies by providing them with more positive images of intellectual disability on the one hand and moral arguments about the ethics of selective abortion on the other (for an overview, see Parens & Asch, 2012). There is a need to approach this issue differently.[3] Much more important than asking what parents ought to do or insisting that state regulations should provide parents with accurate information is to ask *how* prenatal testing governs. Analysis which begins with this question may not be able to help us answer how we, as individuals, should approach testing or how we should act if tests are positive, but it may provide us with an understanding of prenatal testing as a system of power.

Politicising prenatal diagnosis

In her discussion of 'the moralization of politics', Brown (2008:199–200) discusses how the force of history is seen at once as heading in the wrong direction and as being unstoppable. The effect is that history will be moralised *over* rather than seen as a process that can be influenced. Certain actors will be singled out and blamed as manifestations of all that is wrong but unalterable. The situation that Brown depicts on a theoretical level bears important similarities with some aspects of the debates surrounding prenatal diagnosis – as concerns the force of history, which appears to be unstoppable, devoid of visible driving forces, and heading in a direction that hence becomes all too easy to moralise over rather than change. A first step to pin down what resistance against prenatal diagnosis could be, thus, becomes to re-politicise the issue.

To start with, prenatal screening is organised around the fundamental division between norm and pathology. As Vailly (2008:2532) notes, even from their outset, the labels of 'normal' and 'abnormal' have consisted of more than factual circumstances, as they were bound up in attributions of value. This is what Canguilhem (1991:239) alluded to when declaring that the 'norm' is used to 'square and straighten'. As such, the idea of 'normality' establishes a bridge between description and evaluation: 'normalcy' is ostensibly used to describe but also to judge and formulate principles (Hacking, 2007). When viewed in this light, the phrase 'everything looks normal', uttered by the midwife nurse, carries important meaning beyond its immediate effect of reassurance. Not only does this describe the foetus, but it evaluates it against the prior normativity that justified the testing procedure in the first place. Parents are comforted or worried. Further tests may be needed in order to establish normalcy, which is seen as factual circumstance of the foetus.

The division between 'normalcy' and 'pathology' also underpinned 20th-century politics of eugenics. Etymologically, 'eugenics' comes from the Greek for 'good birth' (Gupta, 2007:217), showcasing the idea that 'good births' can be distinguished from 'bad' ones. Twentieth-century policies of eugenics served the purpose of calibrating the population by preventing some people – often poor individuals labelled as 'idiots' or 'imbeciles' – from breeding, whilst encouraging others to reproduce (Gupta, 2007:217). Underpinning these practices were considerations on the quality of the population and the presumption that undesirable groups tended to produce more children (see Pritchard, 2005:82). This was a centralised system of biopolitics which consisted of the active management of human reproduction in order to rid the population of 'defects'. Now, while we easily uncover the operations of power in the politics of about a hundred years ago, the governmental dimension of current prenatal screening often goes undetected. I believe that this is because of the liberal-humanist presumption that individual freedom and power are opposites. Thus, we are not very well prepared to analyse a system which emphasises and enhances individual decision making, in this case of pregnant people, as a system of power. But precisely that, I argue, is what is needed if we are to re-politicise the present system of detecting and erasing intellectual disability.

The central component of how prenatal screening operates as a mode of government is captured by the notion of 'reproductive autonomy', denoting the right of expecting parents to access the best possible information concerning their pregnancy. According to this logic, autonomy increases when people understand the genetic conditions of their future children because it helps them to make a more informed decision concerning whether to go through with the pregnancy. What distinguishes contemporary prenatal screening as a modulation of population management, and what marks its success, is precisely the technology to shape and target the freedom of choice of pregnant individuals. In this way, it is possible to govern without interfering: governmental authorities can manage by shaping fields of action instead of enforcing certain routes of action. This is to say that the efficiency of prenatal diagnosis lies in the fact that it does not intervene in decision making but that the context of decision making is moulded so that termination will often be seen as the preferred option. Obviously, this is not to say that this is the outcome of intentional design, of a malevolent ruler who plans how individual choices should be made. Rather, this is the result of numerous different forces, discourses, and incentives surrounding the individual; it is an underlying logic of a society that favours a specific understanding of cognitive ability and that views intelligence as a defining characteristic of human beings. Provided such societal values and organisation, it happens to be that most pregnancies that show a substantial likelihood of intellectual disability will result in termination.

Accordingly, throughout the processes of prenatal testing, the freedom of individual choice is frequently emphasised concerning whether one should undergo screening in the first place, whether one should go through invasive testing if the screening shows an increased likelihood of a syndrome, and whether the pregnancy should be terminated if the amniocentesis is positive (see Pritchard, 2005:85; Gupta, 2007:225; Buckley & Buckley, 2008:79; García et al., 2008). All the way through, the freedom of parents to decide is absolutely central, as described by disability scholars, in state policies, and in the material of disability organisations. This focus contributes to obscure the forces behind why fewer people with syndromes associated with intellectual disability are born: the causal chain is displaced as the emphasis on 'choice' makes it appear to be the aggregate result of how pregnant individuals decide rather than the outcome of a system that enables and contextualises these choices. In turn, once we recognise this, we must also recognise how parents are encouraged to see themselves in these situations. Here, previous empirical research provides some important clues. Consider, for example, how Kelly (2009:82) argues that screening and testing have become associated with responsible and mature maternal behaviour and how 'responsible parenthood' is linked to ensuring the production of a 'healthy' baby. In this way, reproductive testing technologies appear in a much broader socio-cultural field of 'personal responsibility' for one's pregnancy (Kelly, 2009:93). Along these lines, García et al. (2008:757) have shown that parents often believe they have the 'right to choose' whether the characteristics of their would-be child fit their individual lifestyles. Parenthood turns into a 'personal project', and pregnant people are compelled to see their own life situations and needs as the reasonable starting points for deliberations surrounding prenatal diagnosis (see García et al., 2008). Furthermore, this relates to how screening practices are discursively linked to managing the 'security' of reproduction, checking in on whether everything is running its 'normal' course, and described as a way of having control over the pregnancy

(Kelly, 2009:93; Vanstone & Kinsella, 2010:460). All of these are aspects of the 'field of action' in which the freedom to choose is targeted and exercised.

Now, seeing prenatal diagnosis from this perspective is a way to re-politicise it by understanding it as a system of government. Implicit in many arguments in favour of prenatal diagnosis is the attempt to drive a wedge between state-coerced eugenics and individual choice, arguing that we have moved from a system of power to a system which empowers parents (see Gillon, 1998, in Pritchard, 2005:84). On the contrary, following Foucault's analysis of how power transforms through disruption *and* continuity (2007), I argue that the primary difference between then and now is that two distinct technologies of government are made use of, but to similar ends. Power has transformed to target the freedom of pregnant people rather than use its coercive force to sterilise or in other ways prevent births of people with disabilities. Rather than forcing us to choose in certain ways, diminishing our freedom, we are forced to be free by the construction of a situation in which we are put to decide whether we want to find out about the normalcy of our future child, whether we want that child, whether that child may have a good life, and so forth. Without providing the answer, the technology of prenatal diagnosis raises the question: are these lives worth living? In itself, this question, and the arrangements surrounding it, manages the population.

Now, I believe that an analysis along these lines, helping us see prenatal diagnosis as a question of government rather than a question of ethics, can help us redirect our attention away from individual choices, away from assumed, universal ethical principles, and towards the functioning of power. In turn, such an analysis, of course, carries its own ethos, however, an ethos of critique rather than of de-politicisation.

Ethics, critique, and resistance

'Ethics', as it has been presented in this chapter, may seem like a consolidating, even conservative concept, operating to preserve a certain order by excluding certain kinds of criticism. Of course, the way of understanding 'ethics' that I have criticised here is not the only possible one, but rather a specific discourse that is an effect of the particular modulation of government that surrounds prenatal screening. Just like 'representation' and 'care', 'ethics' may lead to forms of resistance that consolidate the biopolitical regime or that upset it. If the foregoing has been an examination of the dangers of an ethics of resistance, I will now turn to consider the possibilities of re-politicising ethics in order to help us rethink the politics of intellectual disability, as concerns prenatal testing and in general. Indeed, I believe that the politicisation that I attempt to formulate in this chapter – and throughout this book – itself carries a specific ethos. It is therefore appropriate to end this chapter with an extended discussion on how we can rethink ethics in light of the earlier arguments.

Brown (2008:109–10) has pointed out that in much political thinking, there is a preconceived opposition between 'right'/'truth', and 'power'. These are understood as different domains which deal with different things, and their separation explains why the opposition between the political world of power and the ethical world of righteousness recurs throughout the history of philosophy. Brown (2008:110) argues that the moralisation of politics means that political questions become abstracted from the contexts in which they emerge, seemingly calling for answers that are derived from universal principles rather than political mobilisation. This parallels my earlier analysis. Now, one of the great achievements of the post-structural philosophers which I have relied on throughout this book (and which are all, in this sense, successors of Nietzsche) is that they help us approach the relationship between politics and ethics differently from the standard views, seeing that power guarantees and produces moral truth (see Simons, 1995:44).

Consider here Foucault's ethos of permanent critique, which stems from his recognition that 'everything is dangerous' (Foucault, 1984:341), in the sense that even the most well-meaning and positively valued ideas may result in the diminishing of people's possibility to come into being on their own terms. This idea corresponds both to the empirical fact that social forces once activated to emancipate easily slip into becoming tools of repression (see Simons, 1995:86) and to Foucault's epistemological commitments. Because, if there is no vantage point from where the universal good can be accessed, if moral 'truth' is always contingent on *something*, then there is no transcendental point from which our actions can be judged as right or wrong. When Nietzsche (2001 [1882]:120) declared the death of God, this was what he alluded to: a human being left without a universal moral script to follow. The implication for Foucault is that we must attend to critical analysis of whatever functions as our moral guidance, examining its origins, operations, and underlying rationales. In doing this, 'moral truth' can never substitute political struggle, as Brown (2008:106) formulates it, and this is so since moral truth itself is an outcome of power; the reasons why certain choices appear to be justifiable and others do not is that we are always situated in a certain place, at a certain time, and in a certain position. 'Right' and 'wrong' are socially constituted; the struggle over its truth is a struggle over power.

This, however, does not necessarily lead towards the abandonment of ethics as such. To see why, consider Butler's (2005:110) proposition that to theorise subjectivity as inherently political is an act of seeking to dislodge the 'I' from being the *grounds* of ethics and politics to becoming the *problem* of ethics and politics. In contrast to how the 'ethicisation' of prenatal diagnosis relies on an autonomous subject that freely chooses how to act, Butler (2005) argues for an ethos of critical reflection: acknowledging that our identities are always emerging provided a social context does not imply that ethics is impossible but that one ought to relate to one's becoming in an active fashion and that we ought to consider how this social context structures how we relate to others. To use the language of Foucault, regimes of truth, of what is possible and not possible to think and do, offers the terms that make attempts for (partial and incomplete) self-recognition possible, they existed before we emerged and will outlive us. Such regimes of truth affect what will be perceived as a recognisable way of inhabiting the world (Butler, 2005:22). We are not determined, but the regimes of truth become the point of reference for any decisions we subsequently make. Thus, this is a call to exploring how power affects us and to consider the moral truths of our times as contingent on this.

Now, the way we are all embedded by discourses and socially produced frames of recognition obviously has ramifications for how we relate to each other; it is in relationship to such discursive frames that recognition, of others and oneself, takes place. It follows that calling into question a regime of truth means calling into question the truth about oneself (Butler, 2005:23), and indeed also questioning one's ability to tell the truth about oneself; it effectively means questioning one's own ontological status. Hence, viewed in this way, although we cannot author our lives, we can reflect on the social structures on which our becoming is contingent, we can recognise them, and we can resist them.

Taken to heart, this has implications for the politics of intellectual disability. The ethical question of prenatal diagnosis thus transforms from one which pertains to whether the actions of expecting parents are justifiable to a call to understand *why* one thinks of this issue as one does; *why* one sees the prospect of disabled children in a certain way, and *how* the very practice of prenatal diagnosis itself reinforces the continual inscription of the division between 'normalcy' and 'deviancy'. This should be our response to power, to the government of which lives are allowed to come into being; to acknowledge how any choice we are faced with is pre-structured by a society that favours able bodies and brains and to understand how we come into being in relation to the distinction between 'able' and 'disabled'. In this way, recognising the social constitution of subjectivity does not erase the possibility of ethical accountability but provides us with an ethical imperative to understand and navigate the social and discursive conditions of our emergence. Being ethical, provided this perspective, forces us to consider politics by means of critique and to recognise that also ourselves need to be targeted (see Butler, 2005:124).

As alluded to, our social constitution has implications not only for how we relate to ourselves, but also for how we relate to each other. Starting from a reading of Levinas, and expanding on Hegel's notion of recognition, Butler (2005:10) denotes 'the scene of address' the (abstract and fictive) place where subjects come into existence by being recognised as belonging, qualified, and recognisable through how they relate to a set of already established norms. According to Butler (see 1997:25–31; 2004:138–9), 'the scene of address' is a place of judgement as concerns whether other humans conform to such norms and hence also a place of erasure, as not all will qualify. As such, the 'scene of address' is where our discursive exposure, theorised in Chapter 6 as a constituent of our 'double vulnerability', emerges: the place where we recognise each other based on existing categorisations and norms. Accordingly, divisions along the lines of gender, race, and functioning will shape how we are perceived and how we understand ourselves and our fellow human beings; they will be taken as facts about who we are, appearing as natural, yet also being the product of deeply ingrained values of the societies in which we come into being.

In this way, the scene of address is a place of becoming a subject. At the same time, any such act of recognition will concurrently cut off alternative ways of being (Butler, 1997:41); as I am recognised as a 'normal man' (which often seems to be the case), my opportunity to come into being in other ways is effectively precluded. The judgement of pathology, in the same way, rules out normalcy, with an abundance of consequences for one's life course. What I want to suggest, again with Butler and in addition to our responsibility to scrutinise the norms that condition our emergence as subjects, is that we have a responsibility to suspend judgement at the scene of address in order to maintain the openness of the subjectivity of the other (Butler, 2005:44; see Taylor, 2013). Hence, ethics for Butler (2005:44) requires approaching oneself and the other through cessation of the routine procedure in order to avoid the normative violence of calling the other into being by requiring them to exist in a predetermined way. In the context of this chapter, this notion of a critical ethics consists in refusing to take for granted the received wisdom of the separation between 'normalcy' and 'intellectual disability' and to neglect searching for the moral 'truth' about prenatal diagnosis as it is organised along the lines of this division. Indeed, it requires us to stop using 'intellectual disability' as a judgement and to avoid using this label as a restriction of what so-labelled lives can become.

Provided these arguments, prenatal diagnosis is not an ethical question because it requires us to make sound choices grounded in universal and defendable principles but rather because it forces us to reflect on the production and positioning of subjectivity – of ourselves and others. Perhaps it should not be necessary to say this, but I should anyway clearly state that I am not the least interested in condemning whatever choice pregnant people make as concerns scanning and termination. However, I do believe that we all have a responsibility – an ethico-political one at that – to not shy away from asking ourselves some hard questions concerning why we perceive the prospect of a disabled child as we do and to recognise that our choice will be embedded in a culture and society that devalues disabled lives and privileges the abilities of human reason. Re-politicising the ethics of prenatal diagnosis as a strategy of resistance means precisely that: to turn our critical abilities towards how the situation of choice is pre-structured and try to figure out how it could be structured in other ways.

As a more general conclusion to these final three chapters, the notions of 'vulnerability', 'representation', and 'ethics', and the way that they emerge to contest the government of intellectual disability all surface in spaces of openness emerging due to the fact that the government of intellectual disability at the same time both includes and excludes. Viewed in this way, the questions of resistance that I have discussed herein are bound up with *re*-politicisation of intellectual disability, pointing towards a politics that does not take norm/deviancy or inclusion/exclusion for granted. Brown (2008:37) argues that the tension between the particularity of individuals and a collective 'we' – inherent to liberal notions of society, ethics, and citizenship – can only remain as long as the conditions of emergence of subjects remain de-politicised. Thus, we can continue to see the coercive state as the primary vehicle of power only to the extent that we ignore that the 'free' subject is also an effect of power. I believe this speaks to why I have found this whole book important to write: in the end, it can be read as an attempt to politicise the emergence of subjects constituted along the lines of divisions between 'reason' and 'lack of reason', that is, between 'intellectual disability' and 'normal' cognitive functioning. Thinking through the complexities of vulnerability, representation, and the ethics of critique may serve as a starting point to make space for possible worlds in which these distinctions are redundant.

Notes

1 In Swedish media, the new test was quickly labelled 'the Down test', reflecting the fact that Down syndrome is the diagnosis which dominates discussions on prenatal testing, although other syndromes are screened for, as well.
2 For a glimpse at how the general sentiment goes and is reflected in the public debate, see for example the *New York Post* article 'The End of Down Syndrome' (http://nypost.com/2011/11/13/).
3 A clarification: as Taylor (2013) has pointed out, moral philosophy dealing with disability may be important in some contexts, for example in defending welfare entitlements under threat or to argue the case for equal access to society. My arguments here are criticising this way of arguing as concerns prenatal diagnosis specifically, not in general.

Conclusions
Post-institutional critique

I want to use these concluding pages to do two things. First, as dictated by convention, I will summarise and ponder the main conclusions of the book and highlight what I believe to be its main contributions to disability studies and social theory. Secondly, I want to draw on this to formulate a research agenda – to be revised, expanded upon, or criticised by others – of the post-institutional era, ending with a reflection about how we should approach 'difference', among and between human beings and as represented in divisions between 'able' and 'disabled'.

As I showed in Chapter 2, 'intellectual disability' can be seen as the outcome of biopolitics, instituting a division between 'normal' and 'deviant' with respect to the humanist subject. Classification and clinical knowledge of intellectual disability is knowledge which makes governing possible whilst at the same time naturalising intellectual disability so it is seen as existing prior to politics. Provided this analysis, 'intellectual disability' names a diverse assortment of individuals who are rendered a homogenous group by means of scientific knowledge and governmental technologies. This led me to suggest that understandings of intellectual disability often rest on an untenable separation between biology and society. Drawing on Butler's (1993) understanding of the materialisation of bodies, I argued that the intellectually disabled brain comes to matter provided social and political rationalities and discursive framings.

The arguments of the three Chapters in Part II focus on how people with intellectual disabilities are targeted by policies that aim to include the group. Contemporary biopolitics has increasingly come to adhere to modes of government which rely on 'citizenship' and 'inclusion'. When these ideals are projected onto the intellectually disabled subject – a subject interpreted as deficient and lacking, by nature – politics is faced with the dual task of including to make similar whilst upholding the otherness of the group in question in order to protect the humanist subject. 'Otherness' is what citizenship inclusion seeks to erase but necessarily will re-inscribe. Thus, I argue that post-institutionalisation is characterised by the concurrent application of technologies of inclusion and technologies of exclusion, a way of governing that both seeks to nurture the reason and autonomy of individuals to craft citizens and upholds their otherness by surveillance and restraints. Of course, whether the regime of power that I describe can be justified or not, is good or bad, or calls for incremental reform or revolution are all wider debates that must include people with intellectual disabilities as key actors. However, for this discussion to even start, it is necessary to first acknowledge how power operates. This is what I believe that I have done.

In the final three chapters, I discuss how the very friction between inclusion and exclusion provides spaces for resistance. But for resistance to lead beyond the prevailing mode of government and to alter the status of people with intellectual disabilities as the Others of humanist reason, contestations must depart from the ontological underpinnings that produced the exclusion of the group in the first place. My argument here is that the three instances of resistance examined, on the one hand, bear witness to the risk of re-inscription, where resistance merely turns into a confirmation of liberal humanism by demanding access to it, and, on the other hand, to the possibility of a politics of intellectual disability beyond the divisions 'inclusion'/'exclusion' and 'normal'/'deviant'. Departing from the ontological underpinnings of the humanist subject means attending to disability as an expression of our shared vulnerability, to question the dominating modes of representation of the group, and to see this channelized into a political ethics of providing spaces for members of this group to come into being beyond prevailing ideas of what intellectual disability is and implies.

Out of this, I here want to single out two contributions that I believe are of central importance for efforts to understand intellectual disability politics concerning the post-institutional condition and concerning the possibilities of critique. As have been stressed throughout, in the post-institutional era, 'intellectual disability' appears as a contradiction. At the same time people of this group are defined as lacking capacities of citizenship *and* projected to be embraced by citizenship. Now, the simultaneity of inclusion and exclusion indicates that this very binary fails to appropriately capture the politics of intellectual disability. Expanding on Butler's (1993:13) discussion on Irigaray and Derrida, it can be said that the binary of inclusion/exclusion itself excludes the politics of post-institutionalisation, which it simultaneously produces; this way of governing intellectual disability is, to an extent, the result of the lack of a political language that can make it comprehensible, where its structure and efficiency depend on our inability to name it. As it appears, this means that our common terminology is unable to account for post-institutional politics, which I believe implies that we should stop forming critical strategies around master concepts – such as 'citizenship', 'independence', and 'inclusion' – but rather study these very concepts as political effects and as discourses that make possible (and impossible) certain ways of thinking, doing, and being. Rather than calls for liberation through 'citizenship' and condemnations of the remnants of institutionalisation, critique needs to speak a language that does not take for granted the ideals that the politics of inclusion are founded on.

This is saying that my analysis of post-institutionalisation points towards the need for new modes of critique, the topic of the third part of the book. The most central component of this discussion is the development of the notion of 'double vulnerability'. I argued that our shared vulnerability as embodied beings is always made sense of with the aid of social frames of reference, often in ways that seek to project it onto certain Others. The place that Butler (1997) calls 'the scene of address' is where our embodied vulnerability is inserted into socially instituted divisions that will constitute us as either 'normal' or 'deviant'. In this way, recognising individuals as 'doubly vulnerable' challenges the liberal humanist subject of reason: it challenges the norm of full ability, as our embodied vulnerability is seen as a precondition to our lives, and it challenges the idea of self-mastery since our discursive vulnerability points to how we are always displaced by discourses that frame our recognition. Once we start to see ourselves as sharing this openness towards the world, we come to realise that intellectual disability is but one specific modulation coming out of the overlap of society and embodiment and, furthermore, that our abilities are always fluctuating and contingent. Our exposure to discursive frames of interpretation and our exposure as embodied beings necessarily overlap, and this very insight can be used to deconstruct the division between 'disabled' and 'normal', as these vulnerabilities are ontological preconditions of all human beings.

This has some important implications. First, it suggests that we should stop asking whether 'intellectual disability' exists. Rather, questions about the productiveness of power and resistance concern how something comes into existence. Debates on various diagnoses often seem to revolve around questions which concern whether certain diagnoses are 'real' or 'socially constructed'. This way of framing the debate severely underestimates the force of social constitution; indeed, that a diagnosis emerges from a place where biology and social forces are inseparable in no way diminishes its realness. Thus, brought to bear on the endless debates of 'nature versus nurture' and the essence of being human, my argument is distinctively anti-essentialist in the sense that it recognises the constitutive force of the social upon the body (or whatever we project notions of 'human nature' on). However, in doing this, 'double vulnerability' itself becomes an essential aspect of being human; our openness to the world, as biological and socially constituted assemblages of language and matter, may well be what defines us. The ethics of critique, which I discussed at the end of Chapter 8, is a response to this, a way of living the consequences of our exposure to discursive divisions that severely affect our lives. Recognising the social constitution of kinds of people, of intellectual disability and the subject of reason, should urge us to maintain open, as far as possible, the possibility for ourselves and others to come into being beyond this division. Of course, we cannot immediately discard the label of 'intellectual disability' from our social world, but we must ceaselessly continue to question its presumptions and implications in order to unlearn the hierarchical structure that it rests on.

A post-institutional research agenda

Now, which are the implications of all of this? In the introductory chapter, I addressed how much social scientific research on intellectual disability, along with public authorities and international organisations, has come to comprehend of the developmental path of intellectual disability politics as a dark past of state institutionalisation that has been replaced by policies of community living and societal inclusion. As argued there, I believe that this narrative structure hampers our critical appreciation of the present government of the group. In a sense, the arguments of this book have been responses to this description, seeking to trace continuities and discontinuities in technologies of power – *after* inclusion. It shall be restated here that the purpose has not been to deny that the living conditions of people with intellectual disabilities have improved because of the abandonment of state-sanctioned confinement (see Bigby, 2005; Tøssebro, 2005; Clement and Bigby, 2010, 25–7). What I do claim is that we, to a large extent, have been theoretically unprepared to analyse and criticise the post-institutional regime of power, since we have been impeded by this historical narrative of intellectual disability politics as gradual progression. A recurring proposition of this book is that even deeply needed societal changes, including the ones we appropriately label 'emancipation', are tainted with power. The era of post-institutionalisation testifies to precisely this – how something that we in hindsight easily detect as horrendous can give way to something else, a new mode of governing which continues to constrain the lives of people with intellectual disabilities but which we all too easily fail to acknowledge (see Altermark, 2017).

I mentioned in the introduction that the term 'post-institutional' is an allusion to post-colonial theory, which, in similar ways to my analysis, seeks to understand how power lives on, also after we have left the oppression of the past behind us. Hence, it is appropriate to invoke a few theoretical propositions of this intellectual tradition to formulate a research agenda of the post-institutional era. One way of understanding post-colonial studies is as a sustained theoretical effort to complicate the presumed progression inherent to how the history of decolonisation is narrated (see Morton, 2003; Sherry, 2007:11). Spivak argues that historical narratives can serve ideological functions similar to the narration of the history of intellectual disability politics: the self-evident status of the liberal humanism of our contemporary times is produced by reference to a history of grim rule that urges us to engage in an on-going guarding against a haunting past. Thereby, critique of colonialism can work to obscure the production of neo-colonial knowledge, as it places oppression securely in a past that we assumingly have left behind (Spivak, 1999:1). In this way, imageries of the past serve the ideological function of concealing the rule of the present. In parallel to my analysis, to protect our critical sensibilities towards these dangers, Spivak urges us to pay careful attention to how Western dominance was reshaped rather than discarded through continuities as well as discontinuities (see Morton, 2003:123), the same way I have tried to trace how power transformed rather than disappeared with the introduction of citizenship politics.

Following from this, I argue that post-institutional analysis has three main analytical tasks. *First*, like post-colonial theory, post-institutional critique analyses the failure of liberation and the complex traces of how power has transformed rather than disappeared. Again, this amounts to a refusal to take for granted the dichotomies that are currently dominating understandings of disability politics, such as power versus citizenship and inclusion versus exclusion. *Second*, post-institutional analysis attends to how intellectual disability is constituted as an 'otherness' of humanist reason. This means that it becomes worthwhile to question whether the ideals of 'independence', 'citizenship', and 'inclusion' reinforces the worldview that rendered people of this group 'others' in the first place. Furthermore, this also means recognising the role of these ideas in the constitution of medical and psychological knowledge of the condition. *Third*, post-institutional analysis is cautious to view 'intellectual disability' as a fixed category of people with a common interest but rather sees this condition as a political construct that always already bears the marks of power. Nevertheless, it realises that critical efforts that span the divide between people with intellectual disabilities and non-disabled researchers are necessary and valuable. This is saying that post-institutional analysis seeks to *learn how to learn from* rather than *learn about* people with intellectual disabilities.

Answers and approaches that respond to these tasks have only partly been formulated in this book. It is my hope that the future will see more and better efforts to understand the state of intellectual disability politics and its relation to intellectual normalcy – in joint analytical efforts of social theorists and political activists, with and without the label of intellectual disability.

Difference approached differently

Last, remember the short section on research ethics in the introductory chapter? There, I mentioned in passing that the process of writing this book has been one in which I have had to find a vocabulary to put into words my occasional but recurring sense that there is something suspicious going on in the way that I relate to the people with intellectual disabilities that I know. Our interactions are seemingly distorted by structures that lie beyond my grasp but that are still inevitably constitutive of who I am and of the scenes of recognition where we meet. The critical ethos that I described at the end of Chapter 8 relates to this, as it calls upon us to examine the border which separates the other from myself. Now, this state of being unable to give appropriate recognition to others within the present regimes of truth can, as Butler (2005:25) suggests, serve as a starting point for a radical questioning of our present ways of living together. In turn, it appears to me that to approach people who are different from ourselves by seeing what separates us as contingent on social and historical forces is to transform our relationships; when we realise the political stakes of dividing humanity into categories that permeate our interactions, it may instil the humility necessary to abstain from judgement in order to keep open the subjectivity of the other. Critical approaches to social divisions and power are never mere intellectual exercises; interpretation, here and everywhere, serves a purpose and has consequences.

Now, although the arguments of this book were developed with respect to intellectual disability, they are certainly also about the human predicament in general. The implication of a critique of the separation between politics and human nature is that we can neither take difference for granted, as it is politically invested, nor seek to collapse it into common humanity, since that would only create a new master narrative of what humans are. Rather, I believe that we should take the recognition of the socially constituted disabled brain as an impetus to approach difference differently. To approach difference differently is to take socially constituted separations as a starting point for examining what makes and upholds categorisations and hierarchies of human beings, why certain differences appear to us, and what we, as individuals and as a society, invest in them. Confronting difference in this way means moving on from questions regarding the (often biological) causes of difference, towards questions that revolve around the political rationalities and mechanisms which run beneath their constitution. It means recognising that we are all coming into being on either side of the division between 'able' and 'disabled' but also that our lives cannot be captured by such a crude categorisation.

In these concluding pages, I have intended to specify how the act of criticism may be the start of this. More specifically, I believe that criticisms of the divisions separating us – in this context along the lines of 'intelligence' – can be joint efforts undertaken across the divide between 'them' and 'us', where its inherent hierarchical relationship is suspended; perhaps the act of examining what makes us different from each other is a place where, at least temporarily, it becomes possible to be equals? In Chapter 7, I mentioned that the conversation I had with the activists with intellectual disabilities appeared to be a collaborative analytical effort, not undoing the pre-existing hierarchy between researchers and disabled people but certainly messing with it. Thus, one possible future for intellectual disability politics may start in the mutual and critical endeavour of examining why we are separated by historical and social circumstances, why a hierarchy exists, put before us and between us, and to allow ourselves to do this across the very boundaries dividing us.

Appendix

Municipality A

Street-level support workers: AP1–AP15
Managers: AM1–AM5

Municipality B

Street-level support workers: BP1–BP2
Bureaucrats: BB1–BB2
Sheltered employment: BSP1–BSP3

Municipality C

Street-level support workers: CP1–CP5

Municipality D

Street-level support workers: D1

Disability movement

Grunden: Andrea, Olof, Monica, Emma, Anders

Informant interviews

Svenska Downföreningen – Marita Wengelin
FUB – Judith Timoney

References

(AAIDD) American Association of Intellectual and Developmental Disabilities. (2010) *Intellectual Disability: Definition, Classification, and Systems of Supports* (Eleventh Edition). Washington: American Association of Intellectual and Developmental Disabilities.

Acharya, Kruti. (2011) Prenatal Testing for Intellectual Disability: Misperceptions and Reality with Lessons from Down Syndrome. *Developmental Disabilities Research Reviews*, 17:27–31.

Addington, Anjené M. & Rapoport, Judith L. (2012) Annual Research Review: Impact of Advances in Genetics in Understanding Developmental Psychopathology. *Journal of Child Psychology and Psychiatry*, 53(5):510–518.

Altermark, Niklas. (2014) The Ideology of Neuroscience and Intellectual Disability: Reconstituting the 'Disordered' Brain. *Disability & Society*, 29(9):1460–1472.

Altermark, Niklas. (2015) Powers of Classification: Politics and Biology in Understandings of Intellectual Disability. *Review of Disability Studies: An International Journal*, 11(1):68–83.

Altermark, Niklas. (2017) The post-institutional era: visions of history in research on intellectual disability. Disability & Society, ahead of print: DOI: http://dx.doi.org/10.1080/09687599.2017.1322497.

Amundson, Ron & Tresky, Shari. (2007) On a Bioethical Challenge to Disability Rights. *Journal of Medicine and Philosophy*, 32:541–561.

Anderson, Bridget. (2013) *Us and Them? The Dangerous Politics of Immigration Control.* Oxford: Oxford University Press.

Arneil, Barbara. (2009) Disability, Self Image, and Modern Political Theory. *Political Theory*, 37(2):218–242.

Axelsson, Thom. (2007) *Rätt elev i rätt klass. Skola, begåvning och styrning 1910–1950.* Linköping: Linköping Studies in Arts and Science No. 379.

Barnes, Colin. (1996) Disability and the Myth of the Independent Researcher, *Disability & Society*, 11(1):107–110.

Barnes, Colin. (2003) What a Difference a Decade Makes: Reflections on Doing 'Emancipatory' Disability Research, *Disability & Society*, 18(1):3–17.

Barnes, Colin. (2012) Understanding the Social Model of Disability: Past, Present and Future. In Watson, Nick, Roulstone, Alan & Thomas, Carol (Eds.), *Routledge Handbook of Disability Studies*. London: Routledge.

Bennett, Paul. (2006) *Abnormal and Clinical Psychology: An Introductory Textbook* (Second Edition). Maidenhead: Open University Press.

Bernardini, Paola. (2010) Human Dignity and Human Capabilities in Martha C. Nussbaum. *Iustum Aequum Salutare VI*, 4:45–51.

Bhabha, Homi. (2005) Foreword: Framing Fanon. In Fanon, Frantz (Ed.), *The Wretched of the Earth*. New York: Grove Press.

Bigby, Christine. (2005) The Impact of Policy Tensions and Organizational Demands on the Process of Moving Out of an Institution. In Johnson, Kelley & Traustadóttir, Rannveig (Eds.), *Deinstitutionalization and People with Intellectual Disabilities*. London: Jessica Kingsley Publishers.

Binet, Alfred & Simon, Théodore H. (1914) *Mentally Defective Children*. London: Edward Arnold.

Borkowski, John G., Carothers, Shannon S., Howards, Kimberly, Schatz, Julie & Farris, Jocelyn R. (2007) Intellectual Assessment and Intellectual Disability. In Jacobson, John W., Mulick, James A. & Rojahn, Johannes (Eds.), *Handbook of Intellectual and Developmental Disabilities*. New York, NY: Springer.

Borthwick-Duffy, Sharon A. (2007) Adaptive Behavior. In Jacobson, John W., Mulick, James A. & Rojahn, Johannes (Eds.), *Handbook of Intellectual and Developmental Disabilities*. New York, NY: Springer.

Brady, Cheyne. (1865) *The Training of Idiotic and Feeble-Minded Children*. Dublin: Hodges, Smith, and Co.

Brown, Wendy. (1995) *States of Injury: Power and Freedom in Late Modernity*. Princeton, NJ: Princeton University Press.

Brown, Wendy. (2008) *Att vinna framtiden åter*. Stockholm: Atlas.

Buckley, Frank & Buckley, Sue. (2008) Wrongful Deaths and Rightful Lives: Screening for Down Syndrome. *Down Syndrome Research and Practice*, 12(2):79–86.

Butler, Judith. (1990) *Gender Trouble: Feminism and the Subversion of Identity*. London: Routledge.

Butler, Judith. (1993) *Bodies That Matter: On the Discursive Limits of 'Sex'*. New York: Routledge.

Butler, Judith. (1997) *Excitable Speech: A Politics of the Performative*. London: Routledge.

Butler, Judith. (2004) *Precarious Life: The Powers of Mourning and Violence*. London: Verso.

Butler, Judith. (2005) *Giving an Account of Oneself*. New York: Fordham University Press.

Canguilhem, Georges. (1991) *The Normal and the Pathological*. New York: Zone Books.

Carlson, Licia. (2010) *The Faces of Intellectual Disability: Philosophical Reflections*. Bloomington and Indianapolis: Indiana University Press.

Carr, Alan & O'Reilly, Gary. (2007a) Diagnosis, Classification and Epidemiology. In Carr, Alan, O'Reilly, Gary, Noonan Walsh, Patricia & McEvoy, John (Eds.), *The Handbook of Intellectual Disability and Clinical Psychology Practice*. London: Routledge.

Carr, Alan & O'Reilly, Gary. (2007b) Lifespan Development and the Family Lifecycle. In Carr, Alan, O'Reilly, Gary, Noonan Walsh, Patricia & McEvoy, John (Eds.), *The Handbook of Intellectual Disability and Clinical Psychology Practice*. London: Routledge.

Chappel, Anne Louise. (2000) Emergence of Participatory Research in Learning Difficulty Research: Understanding the Context. *British Journal of Learning Disabilities*, 28:38–43.

Claassen, Rutger. (2014) Human Dignity in the Capability Approach. In Düwell, Marcus, Braarvig, Jens, Brownsword, Roger & Mieth, Dietmar (Eds.), *The Cambridge Handbook of Human Dignity*. Cambridge: Cambridge University Press.

Clement, Tim & Bigby, Christine. (2010) *Group Homes for People with Intellectual Disabilities: Encouraging Inclusion and Participation*. London: Jessica Kingsley Publishers.

Clifford Simplican, Stacy. (2015) *The Capacity Contract: Intellectual Disability and the Question of Citizenship*. Minneapolis: University of Minnesota Press.

Clouston, Thomas S. (1883) *Clinical Lectures on Mental Diseases*. London: J. & A. Churchill.

Council of Europe. (2006) *Council of Europe Disability Action Plan 2006–2015*. Rec (2006)5. Accessed on 12 February 2015 from www.coe.int/t/e/social_cohesion/soc%2Dsp/Rec_2006_5%20Disability%20Action%20Plan.pdf.

Cruikshank, Barbara. (1999) *The Will to Empower: Democratic Citizens and Other Subjects*. New York: Cornell University Press.

Cumella, Stuart. (2008) New Public Management and Public Services for People with an Intellectual Disability: A Review of the Implementation of Valuing People in England. *Journal of Policy and Practice in Intellectual Disabilities*, 5(3):178–186.

Daly, Mary. (2006) Social Exclusion as Concept and Policy Template in the European Union. *Center for European Studies Working Paper Series #135*. Belfast: Queens University.

Darwin, Horace, Darwin, Ida, Farrer, K. E., Keynes, Florence A., Whetham, Catherine D. & Whetham, W. C. D. (1909) Preface. In Galton, Francis, Inge, W. R., Pigou, Prof. & Dendy, Mary (Eds.), *The Problem of the Feeble-Minded: An Abstract of the Report of the Royal Commission on the Care and Control of the Feeble-Minded*. London: P. S. King & Son.

Davey, Herbert. (1914) *The Law Relating to the Mentally Defective: The Mental Deficiency Act, 1913* (Second Edition). London: Stevens and Sons, Limited.

Davis, Lennard. (1995) *Enforcing Normalcy: Disability, Deafness, and the Body*. New York: Verso.

Davis, Lennard. (2002) *Bending over Backwards: Disability, Dismodernism, and Other Difficult Positions*. New York: New York University Press.

Deleuze, Gilles. (1992) Postscript on the Societies of Control. *October*, 59:3–7.

Dendy, Walter C. (1853) *A Discourse on the Birth & Pilgrimage of Thought*. London: Longman, Brown, Green, and Longmans.

Department of Health (UK). (2001) Valuing People: A New Strategy for Learning Disability for the 21st Century. Accessed on 1 September 2017 from www.gov.uk/government/uploads/system/uploads/attachment_data/file/250877/5086.pdf

Derrida, Jacques. (1997) *Of Grammatology* (Corrected Edition). Baltimore: The John Hopkins University Press.

Derrida, Jacques. (2001) *Writing and Difference*. London: Routledge.

De Vries, Petrus & Oliver, Chris. (2009) Editorial: Intellectual Disabilities and Genetic Disorders Can Lead the Way in Translational Research. *Journal of Intellectual Disability Research*, 53(10):829–830.

Drake, Robert F. (1999) *Understanding Disability Policies*. London: Macmillan.

Drinkwater, Chris. (2005) Supported Living and the Production of Individuals. In Tremain, Shelley (Ed.), *Foucault and the Government of Disability*. Ann Arbor: The University of Michigan Press.

Ellis, William. (2014) Simulacral, Genealogical, Auratic and Representational Failure: Bushman Authenticity as Methodological Collapse. *Critical Arts*, 28(3):493–520.

Erevelles, Nirmala. (2002) (Im)material Citizens: Cognitive Disability, Race, and the Politics of Citizenship. *Disability, Culture and Education*, 1(1):5–25.

EUROCAT. (2010) *Special Report: Prenatal Screening Policies in Europe*. Newtonabbey: University of Ulster.

European Intellectual Disability Research Network (EIDRN). (2003) *Intellectual Disability in Europe: Working Papers*. Canterbury: University of Kent at Canterbury – Tizard Centre.

Fareld, Victoria. (2008) *Att vara utom sig inom sig: Charles Taylor, erkännandet och Hegels aktualitet*. Göteborg: Glänta.

Fine, Michael. (2004) Renewing the Social Vision of Care. *Australian Journal of Social Issues*, 39(3):217–232.

Flynn, James R. & Widaman, Keith F. (2008) The Flynn Effect and The Shadow of the Past: Mental Retardation and the Indefensible and Indispensible Role of IQ. *International Review of Research in Mental Retardation*, 35:121–149.

Foley, Simon. (2016) Normalisation and Its Discontents: Continuing Conceptual Confusion over Theory/Praxis Issues Regarding the Empowerment of People with Intellectual Disabilities. *Journal of Intellectual and Developmental Disability*, 41(2):177–185.

Foucault, Michel. (1980) *Power/Knowledge: Selected Interviews and Other Writings*. Gordin, C. (Ed.). New York: Pantheon Books.

Foucault, Michel. (1982) The Subject and Power. *Critical Inquiry*, 8(4):777–795.

Foucault, Michel. (1984) On the Genealogy on Ethics: An Overview of Work in Progress. In Rainbow, Paul (Ed.), *The Foucault Reader*. New York: Pantheon.

Foucault, Michel. (1990) *The History of Sexuality: Vol. 1. The Will to Knowledge*. Harmondsworth: Penguin.

Foucault, Michel. (1991) *Discipline and Punish: The Birth of the Prison*. London: Penguin Books.

Foucault, Michel. (1997) *The Politics of Truth*. New York: Semiotext(e).

Foucault, Michel. (2000) The Subject and Power. In Faubion, James D. (Eds.), *Power*. New York: The New Press.

Foucault, Michel. (2007) *Security, Territory, Population: Lectures at the Collège de France 1977–1978*. New York: Palgrave Macmillan.

Foucault, Michel. (2010) *The Government of Self and Others: Lectures at the Collège de France 1982–1983*. New York: Palgrave Macmillan.

Foucault, Michel. (2011) *The Courage of the Truth (The Government of Self and Others II): Lectures at the Collège de France 1983–1984*. New York: Palgrave Macmillan.

(FRA) European Union Agency for Fundamental Rights. (2010) *The Right to Political Participation of Persons with Mental Health Problems and Persons with Intellectual Disabilities*. Vienna: European Union Agency for Fundamental Rights.

(FRA) European Union Agency for Fundamental Rights. (2012) *Choice and Control: The Right to Independent Living: Experiences of Persons with Intellectual Disabilities and Persons with Mental Health Problems in Nine EU Member States*. Vienna: European Agency for Fundamental Rights.

(FRA) European Union Agency for Fundamental Rights. (2013) *Legal Capacity of Persons with Intellectual Disabilities and Persons with Mental Health Problems*. Vienna: European Agency for Fundamental Rights.

Fraser, Nancy & Gordon, Linda. (1997) 'Dependency' Demystified: Inscriptions of Power in a Keyword of the Welfare State. In Pettit, Philip & Goodin, Robert E. (Eds.), *Contemporary Political Philosophy: An Anthology*. Chichester: Wiley.

Fyson, Rachel. & Fox, Liz. (2013) Inclusion or Outcomes? Tensions in the Involvement of People with Learning Disabilities in Strategic Planning. *Disability & Society*, 29(2): 239–254.

Galvin, Rose. (2004) Can Welfare Reform Make Disability Disappear? *Australian Journal of Social Issues*, 39(3):343–355.

García, Elisa, Timmermans, Danielle R. M. & van Leeuwen, Evert. (2008) The Impact of Ethical Beliefs on Decisions about Prenatal Screening Tests: Searching for Justification. *Social Science & Medicine*, 66:753–764.

Garland Thomson, Rosemarie. (1997) *Extraordinary Bodies: Figuring Physical Disability in American Culture and Literature*. New York: Columbia University Press.

Garland Thomson, Rosemarie. (2006) Integrating Disability, Transforming Feminist Theory. In Davis, Lennard (Ed.), *The Disability Studies Reader* (Second Edition). New York: Routledge.

Garland Thomson, Rosemarie. (2012) The Case for Conserving Disability. *Bioethical Inquiry*, 2012(9):339–355.

Gheaus, Anca. (2007) Review of 'Frontiers of Justice: Disability, Nationality and Species Membership'. *Essays in Philosophy: A Biannual Journal*, 8(1), Article 5.

Gilbert, Tony. (2003) Exploring the Dynamics of Power: A Foucauldian Analysis of Care Planning in Learning Disabilities Services. *Nursing Inquiry*, 2003(10):37–46.

Gilligan, Carol. (1982) *In a Different Voice: Psychological Theory and Women's Development*. Cambridge, MA: Harvard University Press.

Goodey, C. F. (2011) *A History of Intelligence and 'Intellectual Disability': The Shaping of Psychology in Early Modern Europe*. Farnham: Ashgate Publishing.

Goodey, C. F. & Stainton, Tim. (2001) Intellectual Disability and the Myth of the Changeling Myth. *Journal of the History of the Behavioural Sciences*, 37(3):223–240.

Goodley, Dan. (2014) *Dis/ability Studies: Theorising Disableism and Ableism*. London: Routledge.

Goodley, Dan. (2017) *Disability Studies: An Interdisciplinary Introduction* (Second Edition). London: Sage Publications.

Goodley, Dan & Runswick-Cole, Katherine. (2014) Becoming Dishuman: Thinking about the Human through Dis/ability. *Discourse*, 37(1):1–15.

Grassman, Eva J., Whitaker, Anna & Larsson, Annika T. (2009) Family as Failure? The Role of Informal Help-Givers to Disabled People in Sweden. *Scandinavian Journal of Disability Research*, 11(1):35–49.

Grunewald, Karl. (2008) *Från Idiot Till Medborgare*. Stockholm: Gothia Förlag.

Gupta, Jyotsna A. (2007) Private and Public Eugenics: Genetic Testing and Screening in India. *Bioethical Inquiry*, 2007(4):217–228.

Gustavsson, Anders. (2004) The Role of Theory in Disability Research: Springboard or Straitjacket. *Scandinavian Journal of Disability Research*, 6(1):55–70.

Hacking, Ian. (1986) Making Up People. In Heller, Thomas C., Sosna, Morton & Wellbery, David E. (Eds.), *Reconstructing Individualism: Autonomy, Individuality and the Self in Western Thought*. Stanford, CA: Stanford University Press.

Hacking, Ian. (2007) Kinds of People: Moving Targets: British Academy Lecture. In Marshall, P. J. (Ed.), *Proceedings of the British Academy, Vol. 151*. Oxford: Oxford University Press.

Hansson, Sara. (2007) *I den goda vårdens namn: Sinnesslövård i 1950-talets Sverige*. Studia Historica Upsaliensia, 229.

Harris, James C. (2006) *Intellectual Disability: Understanding Its Development, Causes, Classification, Evaluation and Treatment*. New York: Oxford University Press.

Hartmann, John. (2003) Power and Resistance in the Later Foucault. Paper presented at the 3rd Annual Meeting of the Foucault Circle, February 28th–March 2nd.

Henderson, Charles Richmond. (1901) *Introduction to the Study of the Dependent, Defective, and Delinquent Classes: And of Their Social Treatment* (Second Edition). Boston: DC Heath and Co, Publishers.

Hettema, Theo L. (2014) Autonomy and Its Vulnerability: Ricoeur's View on Justice as a Contribution to Care Ethics. *Medicine, Health Care and Philosophy*, 19:51–64.

Heyd, David. (1995) Prenatal Diagnosis: Whose Right? *Journal of Medical Ethics*, 21(5): 292–297.

Hill, Michael & Hupe, Peter. (2009) *Implementing Public Policy*. London: Sage Publications.

Holland, Tony. (2013) Editorial: Future Challenges for the Journal of Intellectual Disability Research and for Research in Intellectual Disabilities. *Journal of Intellectual Disability Research*, 57(1): 1–2.

Hollander, Anna. (1999) The Origin of the Normalization Principle in Sweden and Its Impact on Legislation Today. In Flynn, Robert J. & Lemay, Raymond A. (Eds.), *A Quarter-Century of Normalization and Social Role Valorization: Evolution and Impact*. Ottawa: University of Ottawa Press.

Honig, Bonnie. (1993) *Political Theory and the Displacement of Politics*. New York: Cornell University Press.

Hume, David. (1957) *An Inquiry Concerning the Principles of Morals*. Indianapolis: Bobbs-Merrill Educational Publishing.

Hvinden, Bjorn & Johansson, Håkan. (2007) *Citizenship in Nordic Welfare States: Dynamics of Choice, Duties and Participation in a Changing Europe*. London: Routledge.

Isin, Engin. (2009) Citizenship in Flux: The Figure of the Activist Citizen. *Subjectivity*, 29(1):367–388.

Johnson, Kelley & Traustadóttir, Rannveig. (2005) Introduction: In and Out of Institutions. In Johnson, Kelley & Traustadóttir, Rannveig (Eds.), *Deinstitutionalization and People with Intellectual Disabilities*. London: Jessica Kingsley Publishers.

Jordan, Thomas. (2010) Disability, Able-Bodieness, and the Bio-Political Imagination. *Review of Disability Studies: An International Journal*, 9(1):26–38.

Kant, Immanuel. (1991) An Answer to the Question: What Is Enlightenment? In Kant, Immanuel (Ed.), *Political Writings*. Cambridge: Cambridge University Press.

Kant, Immanuel. (2002) *Groundwork for the Metaphysics of Morals*. New Haven: Yale University Press.

Kapoor, Ilan. (2004) Hyper-Self-Reflexive Development? Spivak on Representing the Third World 'Other'. *Third World Quarterly*, 25(4):627–647.

Kaposy, Chris. (2013) A Disability Critique of the New Prenatal Test for Down Syndrome. *Kennedy Institute of Ethics Journal*, 23(4):299–324.

Kelly, Susan E. (2009) Choosing not to Choose: Reproductive Responses of Parents of Children with Genetic Conditions or Impairments. *Sociology of Health & Illness*, 31(1):81–97.

Kelynack, T. N. (Ed.). (1915) *Defective Children*. London: John Bale, Sons & Danielsson, Ltd.

Kittay, Eva F. (2003) When Caring Is Just and Justice Is Caring: Justice and Mental Retardation. In Feder, Eva K. & Feder, Ellen K. (Eds.), *The Subject of Care: Feminist Perspectives on Dependency*. Boston: Rowman & Littlefield Publishers.

Kraepelin, Emil. (1906) *Lectures on Clinical Psychiatry*. London: Baillière, Tindall and Cox.

Kring, Ann M., Davison, Gerald C., Neale, John M. & Johnson, Sheri L. (Eds.). (2007) *Abnormal Psychology* (Tenth Edition). Hoboken, NY: John Wiley & Sons, Inc.

Kristeva, Julia & Herman, Jeanine (trans.). (2010) Liberty, Equality, Fraternity, and . . . Vulnerability. *Women's Studies Quarterly*, 38(1/2):251–268.

Kristiansen, Kristjana. (1999) The Impact of Normalization and Social Role Valorization in Scandinavia. In Flynn, Robert J. & Lemay, Raymond A. (Eds.), *A Quarter-Century of Normalization and Social Role Valorization: Evolution and Impact*. Ottawa: University of Ottawa Press.

Kristiansen, Kristjana, Tøssebro, Jan & Söder, Mårten. (1999) Social Integration in a Welfare State: Research from Norway and Sweden. In Flynn, Robert J. & Lemay, Raymond A. (Eds.), *A Quarter-Century of Normalization and Social Role Valorization: Evolution and Impact*. Ottawa: University of Ottawa Press.

Larsson, Monica. (2008) *Att förverkliga rättigheter genom personlig assistans*. Lund: Lund Dissertations in Social Work nr 32.

Lipsky, Michael. (1980) *Street-Level Bureaucracy: Dilemmas of the Individual in Public Services*. New York: Russell Sage.

Locke, John. (1988) *Two Treatises of Government*. Cambridge: Cambridge University Press.

Mabbett, Deborah. (2004) Transforming Disability into Ability: A Commentary Based on Recent European Research. In Marin, Bernd & Queisser, Monika (Eds.), *Transforming Disability Welfare Policies*. Burlington, VT: Ashgate.

Malabou, Catherine. (2008) *What Should We Do with Our Brain*. New York: Fordham University Press.

Mansell, Jim. (2010) Foreword. In Clement, Tim & Bigby, Christine (Eds.), *Group Homes for People with Intellectual Disabilities: Encouraging Inclusion and Participation*. London: Jessica Kingsley Publishers.

Mansfield, Caroline, Hopfer, Suellen & Marteau, Theresa M. (1999) Termination Rates after Prenatal Diagnosis of Down Syndrome, Spina Bifida, Anencephaly, and Turner and Klinefelter Syndromes: A Systematic Literature Review. *Prenatal Diagnosis*, 19:808–812.

Markell, Patchen. (2003) *Bound by Recognition*. Princeton: Princeton University Press.

Marshall, Thomas H. (1950) Citizenship and Social Class. In Manza, Jeff & Sauder, Michael (Eds.), *Inequality and Society*. New York: W. W. Norton and Co.

Maudsley, Henry. (1873) *Body and Mind: An Inquiry their Connection and Mutual Influence, Specially in Reference to Mental Disorders* (Revised Edition). London: Macmillan and Co.

McClimens, Alex. (2007) Language, Labels and Diagnosis: An Idiot's Guide to Learning Disability. *Journal of Intellectual Disabilities*, 11(3):257–266.

McDermott, Suzanne, Durkin, Maureen S., Schupf, Nicole & Stein, Zena A. (2007) Epidemiology and Etiology of Mental Retardation. In Jacobson, John W., Mulick, James A. & Rojahn, Johannes (Eds.), *Handbook of Intellectual and Developmental Disabilities*. New York, NY: Springer.

McKinnon, Catriona & Hampsher-Monk, Iain. (2000) *Demands of Citizenship*. London: Continuum.

McMahan, Jeff. (1996) Cognitive Disability, Misfortune, and Justice. *Philosophy and Public Affairs*, 25(1):3–35.

McRuer, Robert. (2006) *Crip Theory: Cultural Signs of Queerness and Disability*. New York: New York University Press.

Mercier, Charles A. (1905) *Sanity and Insanity*. London: The Walter Scott Publishing Co, Ltd.

Mill, John Stuart. (2003) *On Liberty*. New Haven: Yale University Press.

Mitchell, David T. & Snyder, Sharon L. (2010) Introduction: Ablenationalism and the Geo-Politics of Disability. *Journal of Literary & Cultural Disability Studies*, 4(2):113–125.

Moriarity, Lana & Dew, Kevin. (2011) The United Nations Convention on the Rights of Persons with Disabilities and Participation in Aotearoa New Zealand. *Disability & Society*, 26(6):683–697.

Morton, Stephen. (2003) *Gayatri Chakravorty Spivak*. London: Routledge.

Mott, F. W. (1914) *Nature and Nurture in Mental Development*. London: John Murray.

Nehring, Wendy M. & Betz, Cecily L. (2007) General Health. In Odom, Samuel L., Horner, Robert H., Snell, Martha E. & Blacher, Jan (Eds.), *Handbook of Developmental Disabilities*. New York: The Guilford Press.

New York Post 11–11–13. The End of Down Syndrome. Accessed on 11 November 2013 from http://nypost.com/2011/11/13/

Nietzsche, Friedrich. (2001) *The Gay Science*. Cambridge: Cambridge University Press.

Nussbaum, Martha C. (2000) *Women and Human Development: The Capabilities Approach.* Cambridge: Cambridge University Press.

Nussbaum, Martha C. (2006) *Frontiers of Justice: Disability, Nationality, Species Membership.* Cambridge: Harvard University Press.

Nussbaum, Martha C. (2011) *Creating Capabilities: The Human Development Approach.* Cambridge, MA: Harvard University Press.

Oliver, Mike. (1996) *Understanding Disability: From Theory to Practice.* London: Macmillan Press.

Oliver, Mike. (2007) Disability Rights and Wrongs. *Disability & Society,* 22(2):230–234.

O'Reilly, Gary & Carr, Alan. (2007) Evaluating Intelligence across the Life-Span: Integrating Theory, Research and Measurement. In Carr, Alan, O'Reilly, Gary, Noonan Walsh, Patricia & McEvoy, John (Eds.), *The Handbook of Intellectual Disability and Clinical Psychology Practice.* London: Routledge.

Parens, Erik & Asch, Adrienne. (2003) Disability Rights Critique of Prenatal Testing: Reflections and Recommendations. *Mental Retardation and Developmental Disabilities Research Reviews,* 9(1):40–47.

Parens, Erik & Asch, Adrienne. (2012) The Disability Rights Critique of Prenatal Genetic Testing: Reflections and Recommendations. In Holland, Stephen (Ed.), *Arguing about Bioethics.* London: Routledge.

Parmeter, Trevor R. (2004) Historical Overview of Applied Research in Intellectual Disabilities: The Foundation Years. In Emerson, Erik, Hatton, Chris, Thompson, Travis, & Parmeter, Trevor R. (Eds.), *The International Handbook of Applied Research in Intellectual Disabilities.* Chichester: John Wiley & Sons Ltd.

Paton, Steward. (1905) *Psychiatry: A Text-Book for Students and Physicians.* London: J. B. Lippincott Company.

Penrose, Lionel S. (1954) *The Biology of Mental Defect.* London: Sidgwick and Jackson Limited.

Pettersen, Tove. (2011) The Ethics of Care: Normative Structures and Empirical Implications. *Health Care Anal,* 2011(19):51–54.

Pritchard, Megan. (2005) Can There Be Such a Thing as a 'Wrongful Birth'? *Disability & Society,* 20(1):81–93.

Prop. 1992/93:159. Stöd och service till vissa funktionshindrade. https://data.riksdagen.se/fil/1B206C4B-E466-473B-AD84-0E1D9C87B719

Race, David. (2007) *Intellectual Disability: Social Approaches.* Maidenhead: Open University Press.

Rapley, Mark. (2004) *The Social Construction of Intellectual Disability.* Cambridge: Cambridge University Press.

Rawls, John. (1971) *A Theory of Justice* (Revised Edition). Cambridge: The Belknap Press of Harvard University Press.

Rawls, John. (1993) *Political Liberalism.* New York: Columbia University Press.

Reiss, Hans S. (1991) Introduction. In Kant, Immanuel (Ed.), *Political Writings.* Cambridge: Cambridge University Press.

Rose, Nikolas. (1993) Government, Authority and Expertise in Advanced Liberalism. *Economy and Society,* 22(3):283–285.

Rose, Nikolas. (1999) *Powers of Freedom: Reframing Political Thought.* Cambridge: Cambridge University Press.

Rose, Nikolas. (2006) *The Politics of Life Itself: Biomedicine, Power and Subjectivity in the Twenty-First Century.* Princeton, NJ: Princeton University Press.

Royle, Nicholas. (2003) *Jacques Derrida.* London: Routledge.

Samuels, Ellen. (2002) Critical Divides: Judith Butler's Body Theory and the Question of Disability. *NWSA Journal*, 14(3):58–76.

Schalock, Robert L. (2004) Adaptive Behavior: Its Conceptualization and Measurement. In Emerson, Erik, Hatton, Chris, Thompson, Travis, & Parmeter, Trevor R. (Eds.), *The International Handbook of Applied Research in Intellectual Disabilities*. Chichester: John Wiley & Sons Ltd.

Schelly, David. (2008) Problems Associated with Choice and Quality of Life for an Individual with Intellectual Disability: A Personal Assistant's Reflexive Ethnography. *Disability & Society*, 23(7):719–732.

Schipper, Karen, Widdershoven, Guy A. M. & Abma, Tineke A. (2011) Citizenship and Autonomy in Acquired Brain Injury. *Nursing Ethics*, 18(4):526–536.

Schulze, Marianne. (2010) *Understanding the UN Convention on the Rights of Persons with Disabilities*. New York: Handicap International.

Scully, Jackie Leach. (2014) Disability and Vulnerability: On Bodies, Dependence, and Power. In Mackenzie, Catriona, Rogers, Wendy & Dodds, Susan (Eds.), *Vulnerability: New Essays in Ethics and Feminist Philosophy*. Oxford: Oxford University Press.

Sevenhuijsen, Selma. (1998) *Citizenship and the Ethics of Care: Feminist Considerations on Justice, Morality and Politics*. London: Routledge.

Sevenhuijsen, Selma. (2003) The Place of Care: The Relevance of the Feminist Ethics of Care for Social Policy. *Feminist Theory*, 4(2):179–197.

Shakespeare, Tom. (2006) *Disability Rights and Wrongs*. London: Routledge.

Sherlock, E. B. (1911) *The Feeble-Minded: A Guide to Study and Practice*. London: Macmillan and Co, Ltd.

Sherry, Mark. (2007) (Post)colonising Disability. *Wagadu*, 4:10–22.

Shettle, R. C. (1869) *A Brief Paper on the Pathology of Insanity*. London: Barcham & Beecroft.

Siebers, Tobin. (2008) *Disability Theory*. Ann Arbor: University of Michigan Press.

Siebers, Tobin. (2010) *Disability Aesthetics*. Ann Arbor: The University of Michigan Press.

Simons, Jon. (1995) *Foucault & the Political*. London: Routledge.

Simons, Maarten & Masschelein, Jan. (2005) Inclusive Education for Exclusive Pupils: A Critical Analysis of the Government of the Exceptional. In Tremain, Shelley (Ed.), *Foucault and the Government of Disability*. Ann Arbor: The University of Michigan Press.

Simpson, Murray K. (2012) Othering Intellectual Disability: Two Models of Classification from the 19th Century. *Theory & Psychology*, 22(5):541–555.

Singer, Peter. (1993) Taking lives: Humans. Accessed on 8 April 2016 from www.utilitarian.net/singer/by/1993–.htm.

Skirton, Heather, Goldsmith, Lesley, Jackson, Leigh, Lewis, Celine & Chitty, Lyn. (2014) Offering Prenatal Diagnostic Tests: European Guidelines for Clinical Practice. *European Journal of Human Genetics*, 22:580–586.

Sleeter, Christine E. (2010) Why Is There Learning Disabilities? A Critical Analysis of the Birth of the Field in Its Social Context. *Disability Studies Quarterly*, 30(2):210–237.

SOU 1990:19. *Handikapp och välfärd*. Stockholm: Allmänna förlaget.

SOU 1991:46. *Handikapp Välfärd Rättvisa*. Stockholm: Allmänna förlaget.

SOU 1992:52. *Ett samhälle för alla*. Stockholm: Allmänna förlaget.

Spivak, Gayatri Chakravorty. (1988) Can the Subaltern Speak? In Nelson, Cary & Grossberg, Lawrence (Eds.), *Marxism and the Interpretation of Culture*. Basingstoke: Macmillan Education.

Spivak, Gayatri Chakravorty. (1999) *A Critique of Postcolonial Reason: Toward a History of the Vanishing Present*. Cambridge, MA: Harvard University Press.

Stiker, Henri-Jacques. (1999) *A History of Disability*. Ann Arbor: The University of Michigan Press.

Stoneman, Zolinda. (2007) Disability Research Methodology: Current Issues and Future Challenges. In Odom, Samuel L., Horner, Robert H., Snell, Martha E. & Blacher, Jan (Eds.), *Handbook of Developmental Disabilities*. New York: The Guilford Press.

sverigesradio.se 10–09–02. Blind man bakbands i flera år på LSS-boende. Accessed on 2 September 2010 from http://sverigesradio.se/sida/artikel.aspx?programid=83&artikel=3974582

svt.se 10–09–01. Malmö–Handikappad man bakbands i 25 år. Accessed on 1 September 2010 from www.svt.se/nyheter/lokalt/skane/malmo-handikappad-man-bakbands-i-25-ar

Sydsvenskan 10–09–01. Funktionshindrad bakbands med strumpa. Accessed on 1 September 2010 from www.sydsvenskan.se/malmo/funktionshindrad-bakbands-med-strumpa/

Sydsvenskan 10–10–06. Nytt fall med fastbunden patient. Accessed on 6 October 2010 from www.sydsvenskan.se/sverige/nytt-fall-med-fastbunden-patient/

Tartaglia, Nicole R., Hansen, Robin L. & Hagerman, Randi J. (2007) Advances in Genetics. In Odom, Samuel L., Horner, Robert H., Snell, Martha E. & Blacher, Jan (Eds.), *Handbook of Developmental Disabilities*. New York: The Guilford Press.

Taylor, Ashley. (2013) 'Lives Worth Living': Theorizing Moral Status and Expressions of Human Life. *Disability Studies Quarterly*, 33(4). Online at http://dsq-sds.org/article/view/3875/3404

Taylor, Charles. (1995) Politics of Recognition. In Gutman (Ed.), Amy, *Multiculturalism*. Princeton, NJ, Princeton University Press.

Terman, Lewis M. (1916) The Uses of Intelligence Tests. Accessed on http://psychclassics.yorku.ca/Terman/terman1.htm

Thomassen, Lasse. (2005) In/Exclusions: Towards Radical Democratic Approach to Exclusion. In Tønder, Lars & Thomassen, Lasse (Eds.), *Radical Democracy: Politics between Abundance and Lack*. Manchester: Manchester University Press.

Tideman, Magnus. (2005) Conquering Life: The Experiences of the First Integrated Generation. In Johnson, Kelley & Traustadóttir, Rannveig (Eds.), *Deinstitutionalization and People with Intellectual Disabilities*. London: Jessica Kingsley Publishers.

Tøssebro, Jan. (2005) Reflections on Living Outside: Continuity and Change in the Life of 'Outsiders'. In Johnson, Kelley & Traustadóttir, Rannveig (Eds.), *Deinstitutionalization and People with Intellectual Disabilities*. London: Jessica Kingsley Publishers.

Tredgold, Alfred F., Durh, M. D., Lond, M. R. C. P. & Edin, F. R. S. (1912) Idiocy: Imbecility: Feeble-Mindedness. In *Early Mental Disease*, The Lancet Extra Numbers, No. 2. London: Wakley & Son.

Tremain, Shelley. (2005) Foucault, Governmentality, and Critical Disability Theory: An Introduction. In Tremain, Shelley (Ed.), *Foucault and the Government of Disability*. Ann Arbor: The University of Michigan Press.

Tronto, Joan C. (1993) *Moral Boundaries: A Political Argument for an Ethic of Care*. London: Routledge.

(UN) United Nations. (1982) *World Programme of Action Concerning Disabled Persons*. Accessed on 1 September 2017 from www.un.org/documents/ga/res/37/a37r052.htm

(UN) United Nations. (2007) *UN Convention on the Rights of Persons with Disabilities*. Accessed on 4 October 2017 from https://www.un.org/development/desa/disabilities/convention-on-the-rights-of-persons-with-disabilities/convention-on-the-rights-of-persons-with-disabilities-2.html

Urla, Jacqueline L. & Terry, Jennifer. (1995) Introduction: Mapping Embodied Deviance. In Urla, Jacqueline & Terry, Jennifer. (Eds.), *Deviant Bodies*. Bloomington and Indianapolis: Indiana University Press.

Vailly, Joëlle. (2008) The Expansion of Abnormality and the Biomedical Norm: Neonatal Screening, Prenatal Diagnosis and Cystic Fibrosis in France. *Social Science & Medicine*, 66:2532–2543.

Vanstone, Meredith & Kinsella, Elizabeth A. (2010) Critical Reflection and Prenatal Screening Public Education Materials: A Metaphoric Textual Analysis. *Reflective Practice: International and Multidisciplinary Perspectives*, 11(4):451–467.

Varga-Dobai, Kinga. (2012) The Relationship of Researcher and Participant in Qualitative Inquiry: From 'Self and Other' Binaries to the Poststructural Feminist Perspective of Subjectivity. *The Qualitative Report*, 17:1–17.

Vehmas, Simo & Mäkelä, Pekka. (2008) A Realist Account of the Ontology of Impairment. *Journal of Medical Ethics*, 34:93–95.

Vehmas, Simo & Watson, Nick. (2014) Moral Wrongs, Disadvantages and Disability: A Critique of Critical Disability Studies. *Disability & Society*, 29(4):638–650.

Verstraete, Pieter. (2007) Towards a Disabled Past: Some preliminary Thoughts about the History of Disability, Governmentality and Experience. *Educational Philosophy and Theory*, 39(1):56–63.

Walmsley, Jan. (2004) Inclusive Learning Disability Research. *British Journal of Learning Disabilities*, 32:65–71.

Walmsley, Jan. (2005) Institutionalization: A Historical Perspective. In Johnson, Kelley & Traustadóttir, Rannveig (Eds.), *Deinstitutionalization and People with Intellectual Disabilities*. London: Jessica Kingsley Publishers.

Webb, Sidney & Webb, Beatrice. (1912) *The Prevention of Destitution*. Special edition presented by the authors to their fellow members of the National Committee for the Prevention of Destitution. Accessed on 1 September 2017 from wellcomelibrary.org.

Wechsler, David. (1952) *The Range of Human Capacities* (Second Edition). Baltimore: The Williams & Wilkins Company.

Wendell, Susan. (2006) Toward a Feminist Theory of Disability. In Davis, Lennard (Ed.), *The Disability Studies Reader* (Second Edition). New York: Routledge.

WHO Europe. (2010) *European Declaration on the Health of Children and Young People with Intellectual Disabilities and Their Families*. EUR/51298/17/6.

WHO Europe. (2012) *Better Health, Better Lives: Research Priorities*. Lancaster: Lancaster University–Centre for Disability Research.

(WHO) World Health Organization. (2011) *World Report on Disability*. Geneva: World Health Organization.

Wolbring, Gregor. (2003) Disability Rights Approach Toward Bioethics? *Journal of Disability Policy Studies*, 14(3):174–180.

Yates, Scott. (2005) Truth, Power, and Ethics in Care Services for People with Learning Difficulties. In Tremain, Shelley (Ed.), *Foucault and the Government of Disability*. Ann Arbor: The University of Michigan Press.

Yates, Scott, Dyson, Simon & Hiles, Dave. (2008) Beyond Normalization and Impairment: Theorizing Subjectivity in Learning Difficulties: Theory and Practice. *Disability & Society*, 23(3):247–258.

Yuval-Davis, Nira. (2007) Women, Citizenship and Difference. *Feminist Review*, 57:4–27.

Žižek, Slavoj. (2006) *How to Read Lacan*. London: Granta Books.

Index

Printed in Great Britain
by Amazon